INCONCEIVABLE

INCONCEIVABLE

HEARTBREAK, BAD DATES AND FINDING SOLO MOTHERHOOD

ALEXANDRA COLLIER

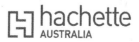
hachette
AUSTRALIA

IMPORTANT NOTE TO READERS: This book details the personal experiences of the author and must not be treated as a substitute for qualified medical advice. Always consult a qualified medical practitioner. Neither the author nor the publisher can be held responsible for any loss or claim arising out of the use, or misuse, of the suggestions made or the failure to take professional advice.

hachette
AUSTRALIA

Published in Australia and New Zealand in 2023
by Hachette Australia
(an imprint of Hachette Australia Pty Limited)
Gadigal Country, Level 17, 207 Kent Street, Sydney, NSW 2000
www.hachette.com.au

Hachette Australia acknowledges and pays our respects to the past, present and future Traditional Owners and Custodians of Country throughout Australia and recognises the continuation of cultural, spiritual and educational practices of Aboriginal and Torres Strait Islander peoples. Our head office is located on the lands of the Gadigal people of the Eora Nation.

A catalogue record for this work is available from the National Library of Australia

ISBN: 978 0 7336 4825 0 (paperback)

Cover design by Alissa Dinallo
Cover image courtesy Shutterstock
Permission to reproduce lyrics to 'Song of a Single Girl' from the musical *Bats* courtesy Simon Denver and Maverick Musicals Pty Ltd
Author photo by Karin Locke
Typeset in Bembo Std by Kirby Jones
Printed and bound in Great Britain by Clays Ltd, Elcograf S.p.A.

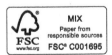

The paper this book is printed on is certified against the Forest Stewardship Council® Standards. McPherson's Printing Group holds FSC® chain of custody certification SA-COC-005379. FSC® promotes environmentally responsible, socially beneficial and economically viable management of the world's forests.

For those of you who have found yourselves living a life
that you never conceived of

Contents

Note:

This is my sticky version of events. It's told mainly through a cis-gendered, straight female lens, but there are many ways to be a woman, a mother and a parent.

I've merged timelines and characters to serve the story and I've changed names and details to protect the innocent and the exes.

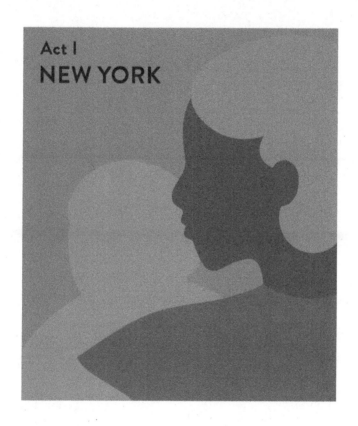

Act I
NEW YORK

Next

I woke pinned to the bed. I could feel the lumpen warmth of Dave beside me without turning over. I registered the shush of cars on the Brooklyn Queens Expressway far off; the stark summer light turning the floorboards flaxen. But I couldn't move.

I'd been carrying around an ultimatum for months and today I would have to toss it like a coin, to see where my life would land.

It was wedding season. Not ours. In 2016, Dave and I spent our weekends and our earnings flying from our home in New York to other cities. We put on our best clothes and faces and made nice with weird relatives. We downed champagne over tables dotted with posy-filled mason jars and filled our bodies with sliders. We cried at speeches and got drunk and danced barefoot on rustic barn floors to 'Billie Jean' and 'Love Shack' and 'Single Ladies'.

Across one of the packed dance floors, the groom, his forehead slicked with sweat, had drunkenly anointed us. 'You two are next,' he yelled as he clapped Dave on the shoulder. I liked a good wedding but the declaration made me want to lie down on the dance floor and let the stilettos and oxfords stomp over my body. Marriage was an institution I could give or take. But the word *next* was freighted with longing. What was next?

Dave and I had been together for four years. On days when I spotted him across the subway car on my way home from work, I still felt elation bubble up my chest.

I'd recognise him anywhere: the flash of his clear, curious eyes behind his glasses; his flannel shirt with a t-shirt underneath; his uncool jeans and sneakers; his neatly trimmed beard that he kept to make him look older than his baby face, topped by his thick mop of sandy hair. He was a North Carolina transplant who said, 'Yes, ma'am,' to me in a southern accent because he knew it turned me on.

I'd left Australia in 2006 to try out New York. I'd first visited as a teenager and I'd been caught up in the delicious rush of the place. I'd vowed to return as an adult. I wanted to be in New York because that was where playwrights were taken seriously. And I wanted to be a serious playwright.

Six years after arriving, I'd inched my way towards my first Off Broadway production. In a fluorescent-lit rehearsal room perched on the windy edge of Manhattan, my gaze had landed on a guy sitting across from me. I waited, as we circled the table doing introductions, to find out who he was.

'Dave. Sound design.' He gave a half-wave, then thought better of it and ducked his head, his eyes sliding off mine.

When rehearsal had ended, I'd fallen into step with Dave as we took the long walk back to the subway at Columbus Circle. We lived on the same train line, only one stop apart. New York friendships were cemented by subway lines.

We sat on the train side by side as it rattled under the East River, our shoulders glancing against each other. Warmth zipped down my arm. I avoided the feeling by talking.

'So, I was just reading this article about how it's important to have a hobby. To be well rounded or whatever,' I said.

'I think I read that too,' he said. 'Or I read the headline anyway.' He glanced at me shyly.

'I read the headline too.' I laughed. 'And it still made me feel guilty. Because I feel like *this* is my entire life. Theatre swallows up all my time.'

He nodded in a way that showed he *really* got it.

I kept talking. 'I mean I'd like to think I'm going to start crocheting but I'm not really, like, the Etsy type.'

He let out a 'Ha!' I felt victorious.

'But it'd be good to do something other than just work ...' I said.

'Let's make a deal. By summer, we'll each have a hobby outside of theatre.' He stuck out his hand and looked straight at me. I pressed my lips together hard, felt the blood vessels crush. We shook on it. By the summer, my only hobby was spending all my spare time with Dave.

I doubted it would go anywhere though. Dave was seven years my junior – then in his mid-twenties to my early thirties. But I liked his Muppety, expressive eyebrows. I liked the way he called me a 'beautiful genius' after reading one of my plays. I liked that he was forever fixing things (stereos and bikes) and making things (cigar box ukuleles and dinners for the two of us). I liked his shrewd, scientific mind.

One night, after we decided to watch a movie as an excuse to lie on his sunken brown couch and kiss for hours – our mouths, our hands, our tongues trying to sync rhythms – I pulled away. 'This is never going to work, you're too young for me.'

What I meant was, *Are you serious about this?* I also sensed a shadowy future where I was a grown-up and would want grown-up things, and he would not. I didn't even think the words. It seemed so far off: *foreverness, babies, home.* I'd never let myself say them aloud. But they were certain. They would happen naturally the way they had for my mother, and hers before her and on and on, tracing along the shoots of our family tree as they curled backwards through our ripe history.

Dave looked at me intently, his glasses slightly fogged from kissing. 'Can I tell you a secret?' he asked. Then he leant over and whispered hot in my ear. 'It is working.'

I believed him.

New York was brimming with a certain kind of person: ambitious and mercurial, always on the make for the next shiny thing. A being bred by the city's unstoppable motion and drive – unwilling to be pinned down or to commit to one person, when fortunes, and romantic forecasts, could change with the wind. In the past I'd been drawn to mercurial types. In my twenties, I'd been in a series of long-term relationships with artists with a touch of the grifter about them: witty charmers with blown-glass egos. Now that I was in my thirties, and still far from home, I craved sturdiness.

Dave was steady and true. He was an introvert who would happily spend hours in a dark theatre replaying a single sound cue. He was a curious nerd. He was as serious about theatre as I was. He was seriously silly. To make me laugh, he danced with his arms in a ridiculous flailing motion or flicked his eyes over my body and pushed his glasses up and down on the bridge of his nose and said, 'Hubba hubba,' like a cartoon character. He unselfconsciously threw his head back in a loud guffaw when he found something funny.

So, after two years, we enfolded our lives, and moved into the third floor of a sunny Brooklyn brownstone with scratched, sloping floorboards. We painted the living room an optimistic shade of lemon cream. Dave built sturdy shelves that spanned the length of one wall and our books were merged, nestled side by side. In the bedroom, our bodies met – our skin moved together and apart too many times to count. In the kitchen, whenever I whirred and worried about the musical I was writing, Dave said, 'Give your anxiety to me,' and I stepped into his arms and exhaled, my body softening and letting go.

Our age gap was never a problem. He was mature. He was present. Life was good. Until I woke up three years into our relationship at thirty-six and knew. I just knew. I wanted to have a baby with him.

Baby Want

I could feel the daylight intensifying outside; the summer heat baking the windows. I had to get up to go to my day job, a commute to a windowless grey cubicle a few blocks from the assault of tourists and neon in Times Square. But I couldn't move. Any minute now, Dave would wake up. But something else was there in bed with us. I called it the Baby Want. Once the Baby Want had taken hold a year ago, it couldn't be unwanted. It wouldn't be dismissed. The Baby Want was a prickling and swelling along the nape of my neck, my hands, my breasts – as though my skin was unpeeling from my bones, straining to get at something that wasn't there. It became stronger with each passing day, with each month as my last good eggs suicided.

My declining fertility had started out as a faint ringing in my ears in my twenties – a sound that would stop as soon as you tried to listen too closely. In my early thirties, it had become like those church bells across the street that woke you briefly on a hungover Sunday morning. At thirty-five, it was a honking car alarm that would jerk me out of sleep in the middle of the night while I pulled my pillow over my ears. Now, at thirty-seven, my fertility was a constant moan, like a grief-stricken whale. It said: *You're running out of time.*

I secretly scrolled the internet to find out how and why my body had become possessed. I found a paper by a Finnish sociologist, Anna Rotkirch, who'd researched the longing for a baby by putting a call out in the national paper for women to write to her. She received more than one hundred letters describing what the Finnish called 'baby fever'. They listed overwhelming symptoms: a 'painful longing in my whole being', being plagued with 'anxiety or sorrow' or feeling like 'a mere empty shell of skin'. The baby fever, Rotkirch found, could be a long-held desire or strike suddenly and surprisingly, like lightning, and was caused by a number of things such as previous pregnancies, falling in love (tick), aging (tick) and seeing your friends get pregnant and have children (tick).

At the beginning I tried to talk myself out of it. What did it even mean to want a baby? It was just the dumb logic of my body. My body fiendishly wanted an Anne Geddes world filled with adorable beings who didn't scream or cry or shit, who continuously napped in mushroom-shaped pillows and tree nooks, peaceful as lambs. What did it mean to want a baby? Surely, it was just about legacy or loneliness or narcissism? Or unfulfilled ambition?

This Baby Want had no place in my life, I reasoned. Some of my artist friends had started to have children and were trying to find a way to slot them into their lives. But New York was a constant churn, a place of unceasing ambition and punishing work schedules. A baby felt like a deviation from that spinning trajectory. Having it all was a bald-faced lie when you were an underpaid female artist. I would have to sacrifice some of my artistic ambitions if I became a mother. That's why my longing felt as archaic and dangerous as being lobotomised – as though the section of my brain that dealt with reason and logic had been extracted.

The Baby Want held no truck with logic. It didn't reason with obstacles – with raising a child in an impossibly designed metropolis where hauling a pram down subway steps was death defying, with my meagre savings or our third-floor walk-up apartment.

It didn't care about the disparate domestic load for women versus their male partners after childbirth, or the staggering lack of maternity leave and government support for mothers in the US. It ignored the blow to women's careers and the indifference to mothers held by artistic institutions. It was blind to existential threats such as human evil or inequity or the planet's climate emergency.

The Baby Want didn't give a shit about any of these obstacles. Most of all, the Baby Want would not be dislodged by the greatest obstacle of all: Dave. Anna Rotkirch had also found in her study that baby fever was exacerbated by obstacles to pregnancy, like fertility issues or a partner who didn't want children (tick).

I'd tried to talk myself out of the Baby Want but I'd finally had to cede to it. It was spiritual in its intensity. A baby felt like pure meaning. A way to create something in the world that was beautiful and real and beloved. Flesh of my flesh. My body was hungry to multiply and make something between Dave and me that was ours alone.

For the last year, Dave and I had been having the same conversation on repeat. In bistros, in the park and, recently, as we walked home from the fleapit cinema at the end of our street. As we made our way down the hill, I grabbed his hand.

'You know, I think you'd make a great dad.'

Dave's shoulders twitched.

'Hm,' he said in a tone that said, *not this, again.*

I hated myself for having to convince him, for sounding so desperate, but I couldn't stop.

'You really would.'

He turned to me, trying to keep his voice even.

'Yeah, but where would we live if we had a baby? We don't have any family in New York and it's not exactly easy here, with a kid.'

'We could go to Australia for a while?'

'But I've built my whole career here ... And I'd need to work full-time if we had a kid –'

'There are theatres in Melbourne. It is *possible* to work there.'

Even as I said it, I knew it would be difficult, next to impossible, for Dave to survive financially in Australia. He had a steadily rising career working on theatre productions in New York and across the country. In Melbourne, the theatre scene was a microcosm of the US. But the Baby Want would say anything to get what it wanted.

'I want to have kids, I do, just not yet,' Dave said, in a way that he hoped would close the conversation.

But when is yet? I thought.

I pulled my hand away and we walked down the street, crunching over the autumn leaves, not speaking.

Dave stopped walking and pulled my body towards him so that I would have to look at his face. 'Hey ... I love you and I want to be with you and we'll figure this out. Together.'

'I love you, too, even though you're an idiot,' I said.

'I might be an idiot, but I'm your idiot.' He grinned.

For months, we looped over and over different versions of the same argument. Each round left me with a clawing and desperate anguish, a fury at being reduced to a powerless cliché: a baby-hungry woman. It felt humiliating, so I didn't tell anyone about our fights or my longing.

Finally, one day Dave suggested we do what all New Yorkers do when faced with a problem: get a therapist.

'How are we supposed to figure this stuff out for ourselves?' he asked.

This was why I loved him. He was a thirty-year-old man who was suggesting we go to therapy. He was taking this seriously.

So in the winter of 2016, we trudged up the hill towards Prospect Park each week, through dirty piles of snow and around dark sheaths of ice on the pavement, to see a counsellor. As we walked to our sessions, a sludge sat in my stomach. Neither of us spoke. We circled a roundabout and stepped through an unassuming door off the street and went up a steep, narrow flight of stairs.

Upstairs, the counsellor, Melanie, was waiting, sitting beneficently on her rocking chair. She had cat's-eye glasses, a whipped peak of grey hair and a linen scarf wafted around her pale neck. We sat opposite her on a brown leather couch, where I clutched a maroon patterned pillow in my lap, my inept barrier against vulnerability. Around us were hanging potted plants and ghoulish Balinese figures on the wall, a Turkish rug and a heavy teak table topped with a waiting tissue box.

We laid out the baby issue while Melanie gazed intently at us. She spoke in a gentle Southern accent.

'I think what each of you need to do …'

She paused. *Here it comes*, I thought, she was going to solve this for us.

'... is find the light within you and let that shine.'

I stared at her, keeping my face impassive as I wondered how long it would take to suffocate someone with a throw pillow. *Stop it. Stay open.*

Like all New Yorkers, I had done therapy for years. I believed everyone could benefit – and should have access to – the talking cure. I'd absorbed the basic theory of psychoanalysis: adults were like dogs with a bone going back to dig up childhood traumas and playing them out on repeat. So, I decided to steer the conversation to the past.

'Dave's parents got divorced so I'm wondering if maybe that's stopping him ...'

I looked at Dave. 'Stopping you ... from committing to the idea of a baby?'

Dave frowned. Before I could continue, Melanie spoke. 'The past is not relevant here.' She swept the last century of psychoanalytic theory away with a wave of her hand. I imagined Freud sitting in the corner, cocking a sceptical eyebrow. *How does that make* you *feel, Freud?*

'You need to help each other shine,' Melanie repeated.

Melanie was, it seemed, less school of psychoanalysis and more school of shine.

She continued softly. 'And whether that's staying together or going your separate ways, I don't know.'

Suddenly I was crying. *Fuck, fuck, fuck.* I was annoyed with myself. I didn't want to be crying in front of this shining hippy on her rocking chair.

Melanie leant forward, and fixed her gaze on me as the rocking chair creaked out a sigh.

'You seem very moved, Ally.'

No shit, I thought.

'What are the tears about?'

Wasn't it fucking obvious? I tried to pull it together to speak. It took a long moment involving a scuffle with the tissue box, while I caught my breath.

'It's just that, if we break up, I'm worried that I'm already in my late thirties and it will be too late. That I won't meet someone to have a family with.'

Melanie furrowed her brow in a way that I hoped meant my fears were unfounded. But what if I did end up alone? Single at thirty-seven, childless and ticking towards forty. My fertility window closing. It wasn't just that I wanted a baby with Dave. I wanted a baby, I realised, full stop. My life would feel half-lived without one.

What if every minute I spent on trying to figure out this question with Dave was wasted time when I should have been looking for someone else to fall in love with, to have a child with?

I'd recently heard an interview with *New York* magazine columnist Alyssa Shelasky who had longed for a baby in her late thirties. She was single, so she'd decided to become a solo mother by choice using donor sperm. I had never heard of the term 'solo mother by choice'. Perhaps there was another way to get what I wanted. A single, emancipated life. But while I admired her bravery, solo motherhood sounded extreme. That would never happen to me.

Melanie nodded along with my worries but provided no reassurance. We left the session without answers.

'I liked her,' Dave said, as he walked me to the subway station.

'I don't know,' I said, trying to conceal my cynicism. 'The shine stuff?'

'Yeah, it was a bit woo-woo but she's probably right,' he said.

'What do you mean?'

'Like, we need to do what makes us happy.' He leant over to kiss me goodbye. 'And you make me happy,' he said.

'You make me happy too,' I said, inhaling the familiar soapy smell of his beard. As I slowly made my way down the icy subway stairs alone, I wondered what the hell he meant. Was he saying that I made him happy and therefore my happiness was important? Or that having a baby would make me happy so he was willing to do that? Or was he saying that we'd be happier going our separate ways?

It is a particular kind of torture being in love with someone who holds the key to what you want for your life and denies you entry to that future. But I kept catching glimmers of hope.

One night, as Dave ran his hand over my body, he said, 'You know the idea of getting you pregnant really turns me on.'

Another day, as we held hands and walked home, he said affectionately, 'You're going to be such a demanding pregnant lady.'

I got annoyed but then reasoned he was constructing a story for us. That he was edging closer to my side of things. I took these statements as unspoken vindication that his unconscious wanted to have a family with me. He just had to overcome his fear of the responsibility of fatherhood, of change, of the lifelong commitment that a baby would signal. He was afraid, that was all.

I was the one feeling anxious though. So I went to see my doctor. In her office, she typed up my symptoms, while I tried to explain my whirring, repetitive thoughts, the prickling up my spine. Again, without warning, I found myself crying.

'My boyfriend doesn't want to have a baby,' I said as though this was the natural explanation for the leak pouring from my face. The doctor stopped typing then pushed her glasses onto her forehead and turned to look at me. She let me catch my breath.

'Look, I know people who have children and people who don't. You can still live a happy life.' Her voice was low and even.

'I know but it's what I really want.'

'Well, why don't you just poke holes in the condoms? Or,' and here she used bunny ears to imply that I would be doing no such thing, 'you could just "go on the pill".'

I stared at my doctor, mouth agape. 'But that would be lying.'

She shrugged, unfazed.

I'd found myself in a circuitous and thoroughly modern situation. I was in a committed relationship with a man I loved. I wanted a baby with that man. The man did not want a baby.

Contraception had freed women's bodies and gifted sex back to them without the fear of pregnancy. In an ideal scenario, both partners should be knowingly, equally responsible for contraception. Which meant that women needed to ask for a man's consent to get pregnant. The man in my case had said no. Which left me with two options: stay and wait and hope that he would change his mind soon. Or leave and try to find someone else to fall in love with who wanted a baby. But the thought of leaving was impossible. When I tried to imagine loving someone else, it felt like reaching out for a steadying hand in the dark, only to find myself falling through endless space.

I was already in love. If Dave loved me *enough*, I privately thought, he would want to have a baby. And in the dark and quiet of the night-time, when I was lying in bed and the anxiety medication the doctor had prescribed was making my heartbeat too fast, I thought: *He doesn't want a life with me. He doesn't love me enough to have our baby.* Or to boil it down: *I am unlovable.* But Dave said that he loved me, he just didn't want a baby. Yet. Which left me right back where I started.

Now, on this summer morning, I saw that it wasn't just wedding season – the ecstatic life of family and togetherness dangled just out of reach – that had me pinned to the bed, unable to move. It was the not knowing what was next. I couldn't wait any longer.

I gazed at Dave's smooth, pale chest rising and falling, his flushed cheeks, the vulnerability of his sleeping body. His eyes blinked open and looked at me expectantly. I took a breath, knowing what I was about to say could never be taken back.

'If you can't do this, you have to tell me now.'

I didn't need to explain. He knew what 'this' meant. *This* was our future together. *This* was our baby. *This* was everything.

There was a long pause where my whole life waited. In that pause was possibility. I watched it unfold: us moving to Melbourne and living in a house with creeping jasmine growing along the fence, me pregnant, the labour, then between us on our bed, a small creature swatting at space with its soft arms and legs. All of it retracted in a blink because Dave was speaking.

'I'm sorry.' He was, I could see it in his crumpled face. 'But I can't go on this journey with you.'

The pain of it was physical – a searing through my sternum to get to the softest, beating part of me. He sat up and turned his back. I slipped out of the bed and numbly walked over to his side. I hugged him. *Unsay it unsay it unsay it unsay it*, my mind chanted. We didn't speak. He let go of me and walked out of the room. I heard the bathroom door shut, the shower being turned on.

While the water was running, I thought, *Go, run*. I shoved some clothes in a bag and fled.

Skyline

At my friends' apartment in Williamsburg where I was now crashing in the spare room, I sat on the couch and stared out the window and waited. For the last week since I'd left my apartment, I'd been expecting a text from Dave filled with regret.

The apartment looked out at the bridges strung across the East River and the expanse of the island of Manhattan. It was one of the world's great views. Each day was a different mood as the fog rolled over the river or sundown blessed the buildings or a thousand blinking windows lit up the night.

I'd moved here ten years ago from Australia because my mantra at twenty-six had been John Updike's take on New York that 'people living anywhere else have to be, in some sense, kidding'.

My life in Melbourne had become flat and predictable. I woke every day under the city's smudged Tupperware sky. Australia was vast but the world I inhabited felt small and cosseted. I'd been gifted everything: an upstanding education at an all-girls' school, a university degree, overseas travel, a writing diploma and then a fairly decent job.

I worked as an editor at Lonely Planet, writing and editing hotel copy for its nascent website. I was that cliché: writing about other places that I'd rather be. The place I most wanted to be was New York City. In New York, I would be a real writer.

I'd had two personalities as a child. There was the solemn watcher, the shy kid at school; the one who sat for hours with a scrapbook and pencil writing stories in my grandparents' backyard, not missing anything the adults did. And there was the performer, loudly singing *Les Mis* or doing an interpretive dance to get my parents' attention.

I lived in an old timey fantasy world fed by watching black-and-white Shirley Temple movies and reading 1950s books about girl detectives. This made me a natural-born fantasist who moved through life with an imaginary spotlight. I'd descend my parents' staircase as though I was Norma Desmond in *Sunset Boulevard*. My mum took me to the theatre and there, sitting on a cushion so I could see the revolving stage, I found the source of my spotlight.

I loved everything about the theatre. I loved its dark and musty four walls; the layers of caked black paint on the walls; the ghosts of gaffer tape marks onstage where other actors had stood; the dust floating in the footlights. I loved the way the actors and the stage manager, and even that guy who played a corpse, were all committed to this game of make-believe. It was life or death; theatre was a religion, and nothing would stop the lights from rising.

At university, I'd auditioned for everything, acted in shows and written and directed my own. But then stepping onstage started to induce a kind of panicky, out-of-body sensation. I didn't know what to do with my hands. I couldn't breathe. So, I started writing plays. Onstage, I'd felt separate from my own body. Writing plays let me step onstage in my mind. Writing, when it rolled, felt transcendent. It filled me with purpose. It was magic.

My first real play after university had won an award that gifted me money for a production. It then ran for a season at a pint-sized theatre in Melbourne's inner north called La Mama (named after New York's famed theatre in the East Village). After that success, I'd eagerly explained to an older mentor that I was thinking of touring the play around Australia. He'd sighed and given me a dispiriting monologue about how hard it was to tour.

I started to notice the jadedness of artists around me, particularly those older than me. My so-called 'lucky country', I was realising, was a place of limited and coveted opportunities for writers. There was a constant lament of how *hard* everything was: to get hired, to get produced, to get paid. A fierce clutch on the rare opportunities that artists had, which stopped them from sharing with others.

I wanted something bigger than home, and New York would be a way to succeed in stratospheric measure. So here I was, in the back seat, as Mum and Dad drove me to catch my flight.

I stared at the back of my mum's blonde cropped hair. She turned to glance at me and I caught a flash of her shrewd, anxious blue eyes. Formidable and generous, my mum was a bleeding heart who worked with refugee babies on weekdays as a GP and wore colourful designer clothes on the weekends. She was a bundle of contradictions who was impossible to impress and I wanted, more than anything, to impress her.

Behind the wheel was my dad, a highly revered liver surgeon. Shy, quiet, generous. A classic second-generation son who had taken his Greek father's hardworking soul and channelled it into a life of ceaseless ardour, a workaholic's anxiety humming underneath the surface of his stoic exterior. This was a man who listened to love ballads on Smooth FM in his car – 'There's no ads!' he justified – but rarely expressed emotions beyond mild irritation.

I listened as they exchanged their shared, foreign medical language. Their conversation went something like this:

'It was a pancreatic tumour and he had episodic hypo-glycaemia,' said Dad as he waited for the lights to change.

'Was it an insulinoma?' asked Mum.

'Highly likely,' said Dad. 'May need a Whipple but hopefully not. Probably do a local resection as they're usually benign.'

'Well that'd be better, less invasive,' Mum said.

As I watched the tufts of yellowed grass streak into a blur along the Tullamarine Highway, my dad addressed me.

'Got your passport?'

'Yep, I have my passport.' I tried to mute my inner teenager. My dad's anxiety peaked around airport travel. He liked to arrive four hours early, even when it wasn't his flight.

'Oh and I weighed your bag,' Dad said. 'It's over the limit, you'll need to take some stuff out.'

My suitcase sat on the seat next to me. Why was he only telling me this now?

As I unzipped my bag and started tossing clothes onto the car floor, my mum shot questions at me. 'Do you know where you'll be staying? Do you have a phone number yet? Or an address? What was the name of that director friend you had in New York? Is she still there?'

'I don't know. I'll call you when I'm there. I'll be fine.' I tossed a flouncy red dress onto the car floor then thought better of it and stuffed it back in my suitcase. I would need a red dress in New York.

At the airport, my parents walked me to the sliding doors of international departures. My mum and dad were rational types who didn't use phrases like *I love you* or *We'll miss you* but it was implied in the way they lingered at the opaque doors transmitting their worry. I was already tripping forward into an unmapped future, with loose plans to do a literary internship at a theatre, but no idea where I would live or even how long I would stay.

We all stood there, behaving as if me leaving to go halfway around the world for an unspecified amount of time was routine. If I was scared, which I was, I didn't show it. If they were sad and worried, which they were, they didn't say it. But I could feel the tug of that eternal line threading us together, pulling at my chest.

'Goodbye, darling, call us when you arrive.' Mum gave me a hug then pulled back to assess me. She gestured at the op-shop woollen number I was wearing. 'That jumper has a hole in it.'

'Be careful of bad people,' Dad said as he pecked me on the cheek. And then I disappeared through those doors with a sense that, like everything that had come before, it would be just fine.

Gnats of New York

Looking across at Manhattan now from my friend's apartment, from the vantage point of my break-up, I could trace my eye along the island to all the coordinates of my last ten years. When I'd first arrived in New York, I was perpetually lost. A decade later, I could map every ridge and corner and belching manhole of the city.

My first job was in the East Village, waitressing at an Australian restaurant where I watched rats streak from cellar to bar every night. Each shift, the twitchy, coked-up owner swayed onto the pulpit of his front step on Avenue C to give me a pep talk, 'I'm an act-ah, I'm a writ-ah, I'm a kung fu guru.' This was, to put it mildly, an exaggeration of his skills. 'I came to this city with nuthin,' he continued. 'I made it and you can too.'

That I could believe. Everyone in New York was filled with want. Ambition roared underneath the city's edifice, like an engine powering its inhabitants. And at twenty-six, I was filled with the requisite naïve optimism you needed to live in this city, with the belief I could be someone too.

Just south of the Australian restaurant, if you ran across the endless lanes of traffic on Houston, was a Lower East Side apartment where a fellow waitress let me crash. After bumping my heavy suitcase up the narrow stairs to her fourth-floor walk-up, I'd found the place stale with July heat and cigarette smoke. I threw open the window and the air conditioner flew out. I grabbed the cord but it snapped and took my breath with it as it plummeted four floors to the ground. I tipped my head out the window to find that the window led to an unpeopled air shaft in the middle of the building so no one, other than a cockroach or two, was harmed.

Best to head north away from that incident. I needed to inch my way up the island to do everything I could to keep my visa current so I could stay past the six months granted to a tourist. West past mad cyclists and jaywalkers and flashes of yellow, those endless cabs on Second Avenue. Past delis on every corner with hospital lighting, dusty shelves and ginger cats then round the corner to my internship at New York Theatre workshop. There I read piles of mediocre plays, while I tried to write better plays after hours. During the day, I sat in the dusty office with its clanking radiators adjoining the famous brick-walled theatre where *Rent* first showed.

To make my own rent, I got on the subway and whooshed further uptown to the nannying job I found on Craigslist. Each day I dragged the family's toy Yorkie down Park Avenue as its arse dribbled shit along the pavement. After the financial crisis hit, the family's landline would ring endlessly each day. It was the banks and the family weren't picking up.

The job was boring me witless. But when I wasn't working or worrying about money, there were nights when New York was all spark and seduction.

My internship got me into shows for free at ramshackle dusty theatres downtown, and velvety seated Broadway theatres, and black holes in Bushwick. There were the endless openings and events and talks, where I stepped into the orbit of luminous people who, back home, were abstract pictures on a dust jacket or faces on a screen. I could see Ilana Glazer and Abbi Jacobson of *Broad City* in conversation just feet away from me onstage. Or find myself ushering at a show and checking tickets handed to me by Matthew Broderick. 'I'm just waiting for my wife before I sit down.' He grinned his Ferris Bueller grin. His wife, a golden, shimmering figure just behind him, was, of course, New York royalty: Sarah Jessica Parker. At a swanky fundraiser in an elegant Upper West Side apartment, I was introduced to a familiar looking face. 'Have we met at the theatre where I work?' I asked. We had not. She was Olympia Dukakis.

At the end of those nights, I got a cab over the Queensboro Bridge and stared back at the smear of city lights. In the morning, in my railroad apartment where the radiators clanked, a rancid cooking smell wafted up the pipes from my neighbour's apartment and my roommates played *Law & Order* on loop, New York felt less seductive and more like a vampire who disappeared at sun-up.

Three years after I arrived in New York, I sent a play to the Brooklyn College Master's program. The play was about an Aussie expat couple who form a love triangle with a sexy, human-sized New York cockroach.

Like me, the character of the woman was in love with the city. She loved the fierce ambition of the place, the wild and endless nights, the conversations with great minds, the stratospheric possibilities, the theatre of the everyday on the streets. The character of her partner, also like me, was homesick. He dreamt of a porthole back to a surf beach in Australia. He walked around with a dizzying out-of-body sensation. He longed for the smell of crushed eucalypt underfoot, the quiet and empty streets of terraced houses at midnight. For Sunday dinners with his parents. He hated the filth and the rats and the extremes of the seasons, the loneliness of the city, the way everyone was jammed together on the streets, beetling to get where they were going and furious if you got in their way.

I got into the graduate program at Brooklyn College. Each week, I travelled to the end of the 2/3 train to the suburbia of Flatbush. There, I found my people, my real friends. Brilliant weirdos obsessed with the outdated art and financial lunacy of writing plays.

Each Tuesday night in our classroom overlooking a grassy quadrangle, a small group of us sat in devotion around a large, scratched wooden table and read our plays aloud. We were taught by Mac Wellman, an avant-garde genius who loved us and our plays like they were his children.

I got a theatre agent who worked in a soaring building on Gramercy; her office had glass walls and gleaming views of the Hudson. I sat underneath the building after our first meeting in Madison Square Park and stared up at it in elation and wonder, thinking I'd finally arrived.

Then there was the production Off Broadway where I met Dave. The show was in the West Village, down a doglegged street at Cherry Lane Theatre. The famed theatre had a bright red door that I pushed open, eager to see him each day. My flaming heart.

After that, there were more months and years where I snaked across every inch of that island to meetings. At the Edison Diner on 47th Street, with its Broadway posters tacked above coffee pots, handwritten signs and ornate columns, I'd met with the literary manager of a renowned Off Broadway theatre company. He gushed about a new play I'd written. The theatre company wanted to produce it in their next season. Could he send it to Ethan Hawke to see if he'd be interested in directing?

I was spat out of the meeting into Times Square, amid the tourists, tooting cars, metallic screech of construction and the hum of a million air conditioners but I was hovering above it all, ecstatic. This was it. Now I'd arrived.

Meanwhile, nothing stayed the same in New York. Everyone was transient. Expat friends would arrive for a season or so and then move home or on to other continents or cities. Each time a friend left, I felt the terrible, lacerating loneliness of New York, of living so far from home.

♈

My expat friend Sam and I always met downtown. I'd head through cobbled streets, into a hidden, speakeasy in Soho then through a nondescript door that revealed a bar filled with leather booths and the sound of old timey jazz sliding up the octave.

I sat in a booth and watched Sam saunter in. She was tall with fairy-floss pink hair, a nose ring and a luminescent dimpled grin. Sam pulled her fabulous shaggy blonde coat close to the nape of her neck and yelled, 'Heeyyyyy,' at the Aussie bartender. She stopped to give him one of her enveloping, warm hugs.

I'd known Sam since I was eighteen. She was kindness incarnate. She had the ability to befriend and charm anyone:

human, animal or lamppost. Sam exuded a calm and confidence borne of being the oldest of four close-knit sisters. She was an adventurer with a keen mind, who was geeky about everything from artificial intelligence to musicals. She had a flair for the dramatic, and a cheeky wit.

Sam had barely been in New York for a year – she had moved here at twenty-seven. She was younger than I was but she was doing New York the smart way. She worked in fashion and beauty in a corporate marketing job, which meant she could afford to dine at the newest East Village bistro or spend a long weekend flying to a coconut-palmed island.

'Hey gaaaaalllll,' Sam said as she arrived at the booth. We hugged. She threw off her coat and we ordered gin fizzes served over carved ice. After they arrived, we got up to speed on our lives.

'So you have to tell me what's happening with the play?' Sam leant forward.

I sighed. 'Well, Ethan has –'

'Ethan?' Sam threw her head back in delight. 'Are you two on a first-name basis now?'

'I wish. We've never even met. Ethan Hawke has decided he wants to direct a Sam Shepard play instead.'

'What, wait? Who's Sam Shepard?'

'Theatre royalty. In his seventies. Old white guy who doesn't need another Off Broadway production.' I tried to smile but the news was still tender. I'd cried for a full subway ride after finding out. Everyone cried on the subway though. That was New York.

I pulled my gin fizz through the straw until it was gone and wished I hadn't because I couldn't afford another. 'Ugh, fuck that,

I'm sorry.' Sam gestured to the bartender to order us more drinks. 'I was so excited for you,' Sam said. She meant it.

'I know,' I said. 'Me too.'

Ten years after I'd arrived, looking across at the view of Manhattan from my friend's apartment, I'd come full circle: crashing at a mate's place. What had all my years in New York amounted to? I'd worked hard. I'd risen before my day job to write plays at 7 am. I'd sweated and begged and fundraised money for my Off Broadway productions. There had been shortlists and residencies and fellowships and shows. None of it was enough. It didn't satiate my ambition or pay my rent. For each achievement, the bar raised a notch and there were more obstacles to clear, more opportunities to be won.

I was starting to suspect that I'd never be a great talent. The artistic world of New York City was a pond. In the middle of the pond were the giant, luminescent fish – the playwrights I saw at parties and openings, surrounded by acolytes. The Ones Who Had Made It. Around those talented creatures in the pond circled the lesser writers: the mites and algae and gnats. I was one of those gnats sucking at the surface of the pond for nutrients – for any crumb of opportunity. All of us gnats were simply feed for the big fish, for the whole ecosystem of the theatre. The gnats kept the system going and growing with our inconsequential readings and indie productions and frenzied hustle, darting this way and that. But we would never miraculously transform into the bigger fish.

A decade after landing in the city, my ambitions as a writer hadn't evaporated. I still wanted to write, to tell stories that reached out to audience members and kissed them on both cheeks. But I had another ambition that ran parallel to being a writer. The Baby Want. I'd started to believe that a baby could be bigger than Broadway. But I needed a man to make a baby and I no longer had one. The man I still loved didn't love me enough to stay with me and have a baby.

I shut my eyes to block out the view of Manhattan and bowed my head to the couch, my body curling inwards, my crying muffled by the cushions. I knew the remorseful text message from Dave would never come. We were finished. It felt like a cudgel between my shoulder blades. I burrowed my head further down into the cushions.

I was interrupted by the bleep and boing of a Skype call. My mum. It was like she knew. I quickly wiped my face and clicked on the green answer button.

'Hi, darling! Are you in the dark? I can't see you.' Her voice was morning bright. She was in the future, in Melbourne, living fourteen hours ahead in a different season, where the wattle was already blooming.

'I'm just … I'm in the living room. I'm at my friends' place,' I said.

I got up and turned on the lamp above the couch which illuminated my swollen face.

'Oh, what are you doing there?' Mum asked.

'Um, I'm, ah, staying here.'

My mum left a beat. Her brow furrowed as she took me in.

'Did something happen with Dave?'

I started to cry, again. 'We broke up.'

'Oh, darling.'

'He just, he doesn't want to have kids and I can't. I can't stay.'

'Oh, I'm sorry, darling.' Her voice was soothing. 'All those long relationships you've had …' she trailed off as though she was lining up all my exes in her mind.

I felt a jolt of annoyance at the back of my neck. Her words implied, or so I thought, that I'd failed to make all my long relationships last. I was angry now and, through my sobs, I spat out words that I hadn't thought through; words I didn't mean.

'It doesn't matter. I'm just going to have a baby on my own.'

I said it flippantly but, as I'd done ever since I was a child, I was testing my mother for a reaction. Her response was swift. 'Women who do that are selfish. They're only thinking about themselves and not the child.'

I gaped, breathless, wounded. She thought I was selfish.

'Children need a mother and a father.' Mum was emphatic.

Instead of responding, I slammed my laptop shut and sobbed harder.

My mother who had a Master's in parent–infant mental health. My mother, whose intellect outmatched my father's, my brothers' and mine. The archaic phrase, *mother knows best* floated into my head. I felt indignant but so often in my life my mother had been right. She always had the right diagnosis when I'd had a fever or a lump or an ache. It was selfish to have a baby on my own. I dismissed the wisp of an idea.

I turned off the lamp and resumed sitting in the dark. I stared again at that iconic view: as the sun left the sky, light seemed to blast from under the buildings and the river, shooting the clouds through with strands of nuclear pink and yellow. I got up and turned on some music for company. Sam Cooke started to sing, and as he did, he brought a memory with him.

Dave dropped the needle onto his favourite Sam Cooke record in our living room. He opened his mouth in cartoonish jubilation, tilted his head to the ceiling, wiggled his fingers and did the twist. I lay across our loveseat, and watched, grinning. Dave pulled me up and into his body. We shimmied together across the floorboards in our socks.

When I was lonely, he was comfort. When my thoughts winged skyward, he stayed rooted. When I was lost, Dave had found me. But now there was no Dave. And there was no baby. We would never have one. The thought was a cold metal vice cinching my heart.

Before the Christmas break, at my office job I gave my plant to a colleague to look after. I was, I told my co-workers, going back to Melbourne. 'Just for a few weeks.'

I surreptitiously cleaned out my office drawers and the files on my computer. I carefully tacked up postcards around my desk at work, under the pretence that I would return. I left the Rilke quote – 'You must change your life' – pinned up, a message to my future cubicle-dweller. Then I flew back to Australia, knowing that I would never live in New York again.

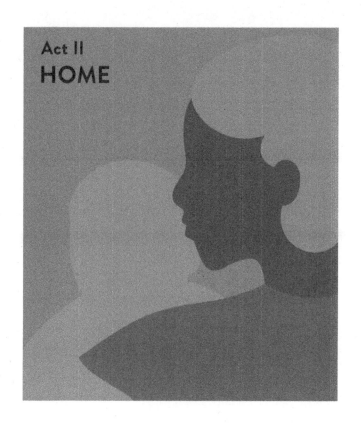

Act II
HOME

Sting in the Tail

'We're going to play a game!' my mother announced on Christmas Day. She stood at the head of the table, her blue eyes glinting, her blonde hair cropped, her short nails manicured in red, wearing a fitted dress splashed with a bright floral pattern. My brothers, father, cousins, aunt and uncle were waiting patiently to eat the prawns, crayfish and oysters in front of us.

Across from my mum sat my brother Nick. I looked at him and widened my eyes in horror at Mum's suggestion. He started to laugh silently, his shoulders shaking. Nick was the middle child. He was two years younger than me but since adulthood had acted like the eldest: steady, kind and considered. He was tall and dark and shared the Mediterranean skin and gruff introversion of my dad. But there was a giggly boy in him that I remembered from childhood, who could still be found if you scratched his top layers away.

'Every Christmas cracker contains a clue,' Mum continued. Next to her sat my youngest brother Tom who had a bemused grin on his face. Tom was twelve years my junior, a lanky 25-year-old with a bumbling demeanour, hunched shoulders, long, peroxided hair that was always falling into his blue eyes. Despite his seeming haplessness, he was keenly intelligent and the funniest of the family, with an understated wit tuned to my exact frequency.

We were sitting in my parents' art deco house, with gleaming white tiled floors and minimalist art. I couldn't be further from the grime and the cockroaches and my life in New York.

'Each clue describes a person sitting at the table,' Mum said. 'You have to guess who the clue is describing. And …' She paused to build the tension and wiggled her eyebrows.

'… the clues are all compliments with a STING in the tail.'

The table laughed uneasily. If they were laughing at my mum, it slid right off her. She was slightly tipsy on bubbles and her good spirits would not be dampened because her firstborn, her only daughter, was home. No one was saying it, but there was a whisper of hope that this time, after ten years of living abroad, I might stay in Melbourne for good.

My parents were over the moon that I was back in Australia. I was happy too, even if I was concealing my grief-ragged edges. I'd lost my appetite after the break-up, and I was whittled down. People kept telling me how good I looked now that my body took up less space, now that heartbreak had hollowed me out. 'It's so strange the way everyone keeps complimenting me,' I told Mum. She nodded with understanding. I was thinner and sadder but I was here. I was home. And I was letting the Australian sun bake me back to wholeness.

The Christmas crackers let out gunshot pops as we yanked them open. We uncrinkled the bright tissue-paper crowns and perched them on our heads as my aunt read the first clue.

'A brilliant green thumb with a stubborn streak.'

Everyone was shrieking and yelling over each other. The answer, of course, was my brother Nick, who was a gardener and notoriously stubborn.

'A real catch unless he's playing computer games,' read my cousin.

Everyone groaned. It was my brother Tom, who had a complicated relationship with video games. We continued around the table. There was only one clue per person but it seemed like there were several compliments with gentle stings that pointed to my mother: 'An incredibly charming woman but you don't want to cross her!' or 'A stylish dresser who can never admit she's wrong.'

One final clue. 'A very talented writer who's lost a lot of weight since last year,' my brother Nick read then frowned. The laughter dropped out. My heart – raw and red – felt like it was pulsing on the surface of my clothes, but I kept my painted smile on.

My family's eyes darted towards me then away and around the table. A line had been crossed. I'd been stung. But this was my mother – loving and tactless and brilliant and biting and always ready with a sting in her tail.

'Mum!' I said, incredulous. She was laughing and saying, 'What?' but it didn't matter because Nick chided her in the kitchen as the plates were cleared, and she said, 'I'm sorry, darling,' for once admitting that she was wrong. Soon we were all giggling again and drinking in the sun outside and eating pavlova, crystals of sugar stuck to our teeth.

Later, we were lying drowsily on the couch drinking tea and I was sneaking spoonfuls of brandied butter in the kitchen. By evening *National Lampoon's Christmas Vacation* was playing on the TV. My dad was laughing at Chevy Chase's expression as the turkey on-screen deflated into a bag of leathery crisped bones. And it was all comforting and familiar and irritating because I was home.

In Melbourne, the summer was a reel of goodness: floating in the sea on a giant tyre at Brighton Baths, squashed together with Lucie, one of my oldest, dearest friends from university.

Short and pale, with a boy-cut of thick dark hair and rosy cheeks, Lucie had a spark in her eye that was always about to spill into hilarity. I loved Lucie because she was happy to overthink everything with me, because she ordered confidently in restaurants, because she devoured food and booze and life. Like all my favourite people, Lucie was perfectly balanced on the spectrum of neurotic to hilarious. She had forked off to a sensible path, becoming a schoolteacher after we finished university while I went to New York, but no matter, we were both single and reunited at last.

Lucie lazily paddled one arm over the edge of the tyre and squinted into the Australian sun. 'So if you met someone now, like your dream person or whatever, your *soulmate* ...' She stressed soulmate with classic Lucie irony.

'Uh huh?' I was curious to see where this was going. I tried to shift back into balance on the tyre, my body leaning against my old friend.

'You would break up with him if he didn't want to have kids?'

I considered the question as I watched a seagull flirting with the wind above us.

'I mean, yeah, I think I would,' I said.

Lucie was ambivalent about having children but I knew that she wasn't judging me. She sat silently, absorbing my answer, then all of sudden, she started to slip off the tyre, wriggling her body to right herself and nudging me off balance. We yelled over each other:

'Ow/You're *pushing* me/You pushed *me*!/I'm slipping!'

Then we both fell into the water, shrieking and laughing.

In the evening, after the sun set, I spent my nights drinking beers at bluestone pubs and having rowdy conversations with familiar strangers and old friends. I rode my bike across the city in the dark, making my way over the bridge strung across the brown-slicked glint of the Yarra River. I spent my mornings swimming, endlessly swimming in the sea and, with each kick, felt my New York sadness froth and ripple away.

I was home. I was thirty-seven and living with my parents but everything was going to be okay. Because there was someone on my horizon. I knew there was. It must be true because people kept saying, 'Don't worry, you'll meet someone.' So I was optimistic. I was looking forward to meeting this someone. I was determined to meet someone.

I signed up for the dating apps: happn and Tinder and Bumble. I overheard my mum's muffled phone conversation through the wall of my parents' bedroom.

'Alexandra's been going through those dating apps, she's *desperate* to meet someone.'

I wasn't annoyed because, in some ways, she was right. Up ahead, the tunnel of my life was narrowing towards forty.

On the other hand, I was annoyed. A woman didn't need a man or a partner or marriage to be made whole. But believing in a woman's independence and self-actualisation outside of coupledom and enacting it were two different things. Love and romance had a siren pull. Not only that, they were a sign of accomplishment – a beloved was a gleaming prize that showed you'd won at adulthood, that conferred you with status and sanctified all your choices. It was rare to hear stories or see examples of women who chose singleness. There was still a stigma to singlehood.

I didn't need a man. And yet. I wanted love. I wanted a baby. Which meant I was reliant on a man. Unless of course I tried to have a baby alone. But I wouldn't need to do that because I was going to meet someone.

That was where the apps came in. There was something thrilling about the apps. All those men trilled away at me, as I matched my way forward. All of those dings and pings and 'Heys' vied for my attention. All those men that I stuffed into my handbag and could check on later when the night was slow and I was feeling restless or lonely or trying to forget the man I still loved who now lived ten thousand miles away. My feelings about Dave had calcified into a scab, a carapace of fury to hide my sadness. *He wasted my fucking time.* But it didn't matter because one of those men on my screen, wedged in my bag between my wallet and my lip balm, might be mine.

I also had a hidden advantage. Before I left New York, I'd started writing for world-renowned relationship therapist Esther Perel. Esther had given wildly successful TED Talks, she'd published books and had a hit podcast. She was beautiful and Belgian and terrifyingly intelligent. Every few weeks, over Skype, Esther's piercing blue eyes appeared in pixelated form on my computer screen then reoriented themselves into her elegant face. She would talk on a subject while I furiously scribbled notes, for Esther's blog, but also for my own life. I wanted her wisdom to transmute me, to heal me, to make me a better person. I was getting a coveted education in relationships from a guru.

'Technology has changed the way we love,' Esther explained in her Belgian accent, enunciating each word and stretching the vowels for emphasis. We were working together on her next blog post about the paradox of choice created by dating apps.

'Our previous model of duty and obligation has shifted to free choice. Now we emphasise individual rights, self-fulfilment, happiness,' she said.

Her brilliant mind outpaced my typing speed. 'Yep, let me just get this down,' I muttered but she continued on.

'We're drowning in cognitive overload ... floundering in the uncertainty and self-doubt that comes with choice.'

I wasn't drowning, though, I was surfing a golden wave. Because at the beginning, the algorithm of the apps delivered the most attractive faces. Square-jawed, tall, hearty-looking men who were the apps' top performers. What I didn't discover until later is that these men had long gone from the app, already enfolded into relationships, while their profiles still floated in the ether. Why? Because removing the app off your screen didn't delete your account, which meant your profile remained. So while I was dreaming of making a perfect match, and a perfect baby, with one of those shiny men, I realised they were probably already married and mortgaged in Boronia with 2.5 kids.

No matter, the possibilities seemed endless. I was about to have what Lucie called a 'purple patch' – a particular post-break-up stage of attractiveness. I was slimmer, more vulnerable and flying on a weird grief high. I was radiating the aura of not-quite-readiness when it came to love. In short, I was catnip to the man-children of Tinder.

Andre

Before my first online date, with a handsome bearded man who worked for the Environmental Protection Agency, I was nervous. Lucie came over armed with a box of jewellery to accessorise with and concealer to cover a pus-filled pimple that had risen overnight, like a Mount Vesuvius on my chin. We were giggling as she helped me get ready, while coordinating my outfit as seriously as a UN summit.

Lucie left and I tried to quiet my anxiety with a few tokes of a joint, which I smoked furtively in a recessed entryway to a neighbouring house on my parents' street. On the tram, golden hour melted over the buildings, the streets were pulsing with light and bicycles and people and I was in love with the city. In the bar I was flying: chatting to the DJ and the barman and anyone who made eye contact.

I heard someone say my name. I turned to find a man standing behind me in a business suit. Andre smiled at me with familiarity. I instantly regretted being stoned. Andre was that beardy type of good looking with an almost perfect jaw and glinting eyes that were shrewd but managed to undress you at the same time. He looked like he could start a campfire in a rainstorm. Like he could bring you to orgasm in three minutes. Like he could ride a cargo bike towing our three beautiful kids on the back. He was handsome, not just internet handsome, and now I was feeling unhinged.

I said hi to Andre, suddenly breathless, mouth dry and stepped over for an awkward kiss on the cheek hello. 'Hey, this is weird, isn't it? I mean it's not weird but there's no smooth way to identify a stranger really, is there? I asked three different people if they were you, before you got here. Only one of them pretended to be you.' I was babbling.

'Where is he? I'll kill him for trying to steal my date,' Andre joked, looking around the bar. Was he flirting, already? Could he be the father of my child? He turned back to me. 'Can I get you a drink?'

As the bar crowded with people, and the volume rose, and other first dates came and went, we talked without pause. We leapt past small talk and traversed through ideas and life and what we wanted from our existence. I was gesticulating wildly as we moved from one drink to three.

When Andre talked, I heard a gameshow soundtrack in my head keeping score. Andre asked thoughtful questions and held eye contact. Ding! Andre asked about my writing. Ding! Andre told me he loved the work of playwright Samuel Beckett. Ding! Ding! Ding!

'So ... New York, huh? Why would you ever leave New York?' he asked. The gameshow soundtrack faded into the background. Suddenly I was back on a subway car. It was magic hour, the industrial wasteland of Gowanus glowed through the train windows. And there, at the other end of the carriage, his body backlit, his head bent over a book, was Dave. He looked up and caught sight of me and grinned. *No, no, no.* The truth was too painful. I fixed my eyes on Andre.

'Um, I think my ambitions in New York were starting to eat away at me,' I said. 'I was ready to come home, really. I kind of fell out of love with the city. I dunno. Sorry, I'm rambling … are you ambitious?'

An awkward segue but Andre went with it. He furrowed his handsome face and thought about it. 'I'm ambitious in terms of the biosphere, like … Changing the biosphere.' I was back in the present, charmed by Andre, by his talk of biosphere and Beckett. He was smart. Ding! He was gainfully employed in a noble environment-related profession. Ding and ding! He had a smile that made my insides quiver. Ding! At the end of the night, on Swanston Street as drunk people reeled past under the fluorescent lights of the 7-Eleven, he hugged me firmly and we agreed to meet again.

This online dating thing was going to be easy, I thought, as I tripped my way home. I'd struck gold my first time; my prize was within reach. Of course, I couldn't be entirely sure because I'd been known to mistake a buzz for attraction in the past but, next time, I'd be sober as a judge.

⚕

The next time we met for dinner at a pizza restaurant just north of the city in a suburb crammed with Italian restaurants. Andre was wearing a retro tartan suit.

'I get a lot of compliments when I wear this suit,' he said.

'It's great!' I said. It wasn't.

But the high of the first date was carrying me forward, and I told myself poor sartorial choices were not fundamental to a person's soul. What did it matter when I was getting tipsier by the minute? Andre paid for the meal. 'Don't worry, you can get the next dinner.' His hand rested on my arm briefly. *He wants to see me again.*

We talked our way down the street and around the corner to a nautically themed bar, with antique ship helms on the wall and red paper lanterns that bathed our skin pink. We were drinking cocktails now and I was listening intently as he talked, parsing his conversation for clues as to who he truly was.

'So how many online dates have you been on this week?' It was a joke but also a test.

'This is my third one tonight,' he deadpanned. 'Nah,' he continued, 'I've actually been having a bit of a break. The whole online dating thing feels like it's turned us into a supermarket of humans. We're like discardable objects.' He was staring into my eyes. I looked away, nervous.

'But don't you think it widens the circle of people we can meet?' I replied. 'Like it gives us access to people we *might* have met, like friends of friends, but they were just one circle out of reach or whatever. Esther Perel says –'

I dropped Esther into the conversation casually 1) to test whether Andre knew who she was (which would indicate he had some relationship savvy) and 2) so I could mention I worked for her and make myself seem more attractive.

'Wait, Esther Perel the therapist?' Ding!

'Yeah, I write for her blog.'

'Wow. That's pretty hot.'

You're pretty hot, I thought.

He leant closer to me. 'Sorry, I interrupted you, what does Esther say?'

'Esther says that, you know, it used to be our grandmother or whatever in the village that set us up with our partners but now that we live in large cities, online dating is like our yenta – it widens the circle of possibility.'

'You haven't been on the apps for very long,' Andre said darkly.

'Oh no, should I be worried?' I cocked my head and we looked at each other. His hand moved onto my knee, making my neurons fizz.

'Absolutely. There's a lot of weirdos out there who'll be chasing you because you're very, very attractive.'

Before I could respond, he was kissing me. It felt odd to kiss a stranger. A not-Dave stranger. Dave. I quickly swallowed down an ache and closed my eyes. A stranger's lips. A stranger's taste. A stranger's smell. Woodsmoke. Burnt orange. Acid sweet from tongue to clit.

There was more slow and tantalising kissing in the bar and my hand gripping the bicep curl I could feel beneath the starch of his shirt and his finger running a seam up my inner thigh, and then even more kissing in a car on the way back to his place. We clattered into his house, drunk, giggling. We bypassed the living room and went straight into his bedroom. It was neat and sparse – a futon with a grey duvet, a poster of *2001: A Space Odyssey* on the wall, Ikea drawers. I squinted to overlook the personality-less décor that made Andre seem less mature somehow.

He was undressing me on his beige sheets. I'd told myself I wouldn't go home with him but, oh well, here I was. It felt almost dutiful – something to get out of the way. We unbuttoned each other's clothes and he unpeeled my jeans, while I tried to keep a pretence of sexiness, even as he had to yank them over my ankles.

After he'd taken off my underwear, he asked, 'Do we need to use a condom?'

'Yes, yes we do,' I said.

Something flickered across his face, which might have been annoyance but he hid it well as he fished around in a drawer and I heard the crinkle of a wrapper, and watched his look of concentration as he slid the condom on. Then he got on top of me and there was that strange and lovely breach of a stranger inside me. He was heavier, his body weight was different, pressing me to the bed, his skin felt different, his rhythm was different.

Within seconds he'd accelerated and was thrusting at a frantic pace, flesh slapping hard on flesh. I glanced at his face, sweat was forming on his forehead. He pressed one of my hands down on the bed. His chin jutted upwards to the ceiling, he seemed to be somewhere else altogether. 'Can you, um … slow down?' I tried to keep my voice light. 'Oh sure, sorry.' He glanced at me, and slowed down. But then he quickly picked up the pounding pace again.

Amid the pounding, I felt a slipperiness. A shock. Where was the condom? He was making grunting sounds of pleasure. I put my hands on his shoulder, half-shoving him away. 'Wait, stop!'

He rolled off me. 'I was wondering why it felt so good,' he panted, lying on his back.

'Do you want to get another condom?' I asked. Surely this bad sex could be turned around, salvaged.

Andre sighed. 'I don't think it's going to happen if we do. Condoms just really turn me off.'

'Well, I'm not on the pill so … I can't.'

A long silence ran down the bed, along the inches between us.

'I mean, obviously, we need to use condoms.' I raised my eyebrows trying for charming.

'I don't know what to tell you. They don't work for me.' His voice was clipped like this was somehow my fault.

I was trapped. His irritation had closed him off so that this was no longer a conversation. I could hardly state the myriad obvious reasons that condoms were necessary without it coming off like a lecture. Despite wanting a baby so badly it hurt, I didn't want a child with a near-stranger. I wanted to get to know him. I wanted to find the kind of love I'd had with Dave. Dave. His name made me feel tired and hazy with booze. So I said nothing and closed my eyes. Andre switched off the light and we both turned over. I tried to sleep but my mind was freeze framing and replaying what had happened.

Halfway through the night, I woke to find Andre holding me, his arm gently circled my waist. I lay there, thinking, *Oh well, the sex can get better*. After all, it was just the first time. Like Esther said, sex was something that you had to work on with someone else, it didn't just happen right away.

A few days later, I texted Andre to thank him for dinner. I was sure whatever awkwardness we'd had was just the usual glitches of early dating. There was so much good, so much potential between us. I glanced at my phone every hour. There was no response. The hours multiplied into a day and then another day, which became a week, then two. Every feeling I'd submerged about Dave crested and broke over me in a wave of failure and wretchedness, threatening to drag me under.

I was just someone Andre had met online who could be deleted. The intimacy we shared, two people who'd been physically and emotionally naked together, could be erased as simply as a WhatsApp thread swiped into the nothingness of the internet. The thrilling apps with their endless humans and their dinging and matching had been revealed as a perilous place; not to be trusted.

Wrong

Four months after I moved back to Melbourne, summer turned to autumn and crisp elm leaves clogged the street gutters. I was driving to a dentist appointment when I glimpsed a woman on the footpath. I'd been friends with her in my twenties but hadn't seen her in the decades since. There she was, a memory standing on a street corner, with her unmistakeable pale face and thick black–brown hair. The same but with a crucial difference. She had a stroller in front of her and she was dipping her dark head like a bird's beak up and down, talking to her child, as I glided by.

Seeing this woman with her child felt as if someone was wedging their fingers in between my ribs, prising them apart. After my appointment, where I found out it would cost me far more thousands than I had in my bank account to extract my wisdom teeth, I sat in the car and cried. Everyone else had found partners and made families. Even if they faced expensive dental surgery, they had another person they could share the burden with. Which begged the question: What was wrong with me?

Because isn't that what everyone secretly suspected of us single people – that there must be something wrong with us? That we were plagued by some psychological defect, some loneliness that repelled – like an invisible electric fence that kept others away?

There was a whole self-help industry built on the idea that I just needed to love myself. Once I exuded this aura of self-reliance, I would find my soulmate. I just needed to go to a wellness retreat to learn self-love or do a course online (*Manifest your soulmate in just thirty days for only $39.95!*).

By this logic, everyone else who had found love and partnership were self-actualised human beings. Or was it a chicken and egg situation? Finding someone to love made you more lovable. And the more loved you were, the greater your lovability. Then the inverse was also true, the more single you stayed, the less lovable you were. The longer you were alone, the more the shine wore off you.

When I arrived home, I slumped onto a stool at my parents' kitchen bench and picked at a bowl of grapes. My mum appeared.

'You need to cut off a neat bunch, with scissors, you're making a mess.' She indicated the grapes then saw my pale, blotchy face. 'What's wrong, darling?'

I told her the simple version: that I felt like a failure for not having enough money to pay for my wisdom teeth.

'Well, you've been living overseas for a decade in New York. If you had a job and a life here, you would have been able to afford it.'

I nodded, grateful.

'And if you had a partner, it'd be easier financially,' she said. 'And you know, people are less anxious when they're in a relationship.'

'So how does that explain you?' I asked.

'Good point.' She laughed.

My mum and I traded in these kinds of conversational barbs all the time, as though it was nothing, but I secretly wondered if she was right. Would a relationship, the right relationship, bring me untold happiness, and erase my anxious self?

For a split-second, an image flashed of Dave enfolding me.

'Give your anxiety to me,' he said.

I shook the memory away.

I could have been in a relationship if I'd wanted to be. I could still be with Dave, if I'd agreed not to have children. I could probably be with Andre, if I was willing to have mediocre, unprotected sex. Maybe my standards were just too high?

Later, on Skype, I waited for Esther's face to appear on the screen for a meeting.

'Haa-llo! Okay, I don't have long,' she said by way of greeting. Her face briefly glitched then unfroze. I had some pitches prepared. I started with a recent celebrity gaffe that could be spun into a story about forgiveness between couples. 'No,' she said. 'I don't want to do something that is in the news for five minutes and then it disappears.' Esther was formidable. I swallowed my nerves and tried something else.

'How about someone who keeps finding flaws in the people they're dating?' I asked her. Esther looked at me, and when Esther looked at you, she saw your soul. She knew I was speaking about myself under the guise of it being relevant for the blog.

'That's a defensive mechanism,' she explained. 'It's a way of avoiding being rejected.' She was right. I felt myself flush. My singleness was my own fault. I pushed others away by finding fault in them first.

But the thesis, that something was wrong with me and other single people, was flawed. Many of my single friends had achieved (and it is viewed as an achievement) significant long-term relationships. And so had I. There'd been peaks and troughs in our romantic landscapes. There'd been plateaus of long-term commitment, blissful solo rest stops, and valleys of aloneness. Was being single really so bad? Weren't there undisputed freedoms of a single life?

What if I was single not because there was something wrong with me but because I hadn't met someone who felt right? But when would it feel right? It had felt right with Dave. Maybe I'd been wrong about it feeling right. And how long would it take to feel right again? How long could I wait before I became infertile, and a family was impossible?

I thought of Alyssa Shelasky, the solo mum by choice that I'd heard interviewed. Attractive and urbane, Shelasky disproved the *something wrong* thesis. She bragged that being single and pregnant had been a real 'panty dropper' for men. She'd made her independence seem cool and attainable. There was absolutely nothing wrong with me, she telegraphed. Her arrival at singleness was a fluke, not a failure.

But now that I was in Shelasky's position – single and childless in my late thirties – having a child on my own still appeared to be a last resort. It seemed impossible to deliberately take on motherhood solo: tough and exhausting and lonely.

I couldn't shake what my mum had said after I broke up with Dave and floated the idea of getting pregnant as a single parent. 'Women who do that are selfish. They're only thinking about themselves and not the child.'

After that conversation with Mum, I'd shelved the idea of solo motherhood. Her words had pressed into an old wound. I didn't want to be selfish, whatever that meant, even if I didn't entirely agree with the notion. After all, no one had a baby out of altruism.

I wanted to make a baby with a man I loved, who also loved me. I wanted a man to knead my lower back as contractions rippled through my body. I wanted to give birth and stare down into the squished face of our newborn then across at *him*, the man whose body had made this being with me. I wanted to watch as our baby learnt to hold up her wobbly head, then sit, then worm her way across the floor and stand and walk and gurgle and talk – and feel shared pride, that shared glance of wonder over her head.

Choosing to parent on my own, using donor sperm, meant I would never have that. I would never have a romantic partnership that led to a biological connection with the father of my child. My child, too, may never have a connection with her father.

These were things I'd been told to want, to dream of, to long for. They were presented to me as the pinnacle of womanhood – to be chosen and loved by a man and to procreate. Even as I scoffed at the archaic notion of a woman being plucked like a spring bud by a man so that she could finally bloom, I still wanted that pinnacle and what attended it: a house full of children and laughter and togetherness.

Was I wrong to want this? Was I right? Where was the line between desiring companionship and bowing to the expectation that I should couple up? Wrongly or rightly, I still believed it would happen, that it was only a matter of time.

Shake it Off

'I've got one for you,' Lucie said. 'I've got a "too picky".' We were sitting in the window of our favourite Japanese restaurant just north of the city, watching an eclectic stream of tattoos and hijabs and oversized glasses pass by.

'Ohhhh tell me,' I said.

Lucie and I liked to store up the times that people told us that we or another woman they knew was single because she was 'too picky'.

'You are going to really appreciate this,' Lucie said, her eyes glinting with a good story.

'Can't wait,' I said through a mouthful of rice.

'So I was telling my colleague and her husband at this work thing the other night about dating the winemaker,' she said.

'Hang on, was the winemaker the one with halitosis or the agoraphobic?'

Lucie shook her head. 'No, he was the one who'd been messaging me for months and then I find out after a few dates that his wife – so called "ex-wife" – is six months pregnant with his baby.'

I dragged my palm over my eyes in recognition. 'Oh yeah, that guy.'

'Anyway, I'm telling my colleague and her husband the story because they're boring and they need to live vicariously through my dating life. And the husband says, and he's dead serious: "Lucie, you girls really need to lower your standards." LOWER YOUR STANDARDS. LOWER. YOUR. STANDARDS.' Lucie's voice boomed across the tiny restaurant. A couple turned to look at us but neither of us cared.

'He did NOT say that.' My indignance was gleeful. This was the reward, I thought, for being single. That Lucie and I had each other.

'He ABSOLUTELY did. Which makes sense because my colleague is incredible and her husband is sooooo average. She definitely had to lower her standards for him.'

'Ugh, typical,' I said. We both stared out the window in disbelief.

Lucie sighed. 'I mean I am picky but that's because, at this point, my life is good, if someone is going to come along, they'd better add something to my life. It's not like I need a relationship, but I'd like one, you know?'

'I actually feel like I'm not being picky,' I said. 'Those married people have no idea what we're dealing with out there.'

'No idea,' Lucie agreed.

After Andre, I'd waded out into the sea of dating options online. Meanwhile, other men from my past started reappearing. Boys I went to university with who were now middle-aged lawyers and comedians and writers sent me messages online, as though there'd been no break in the almost two decades since I'd last seen them.

These men and I compared our dating war stories and online dramas – there was an intimacy to our relationships because there was a complete lack of stakes. We weren't interested in each other. But we were useful bench warmers to boost each other's ego with a late-night text fest, a lacklustre volley of flirting.

This should have been flattering. But all of our contemporaries had coupled up. It felt like we were the last ones left at the dance, lingering by the walls, clutching our wilting corsages, watching the pairs blossom into their future with children and mortgages.

I decided to approach most of these I-used-to-know-you guys with openness. We'd all heard the old, 'It's so weird, I hadn't seen him/her/them since high school, when they were just that smelly weirdo in a Hole band t-shirt, and then we bumped into each other and fell in love' stories. I could be one of those people who fell in love with a former Courtney Love fan. Time was ticking and I couldn't, and didn't, rule them out.

⚇

A year before I returned home, my friend Sam had moved to Melbourne from New York too. She was also dating with dedication – both men and women. We decided to host a singles party at a house I was subletting. Sam brought along her coterie of attractive and hilarious friends who each had to bring a single person with them.

At 1 am, as 'Shake It Off' was cranking inside, Sam and I stood on the balcony and exhaled a joint into the cold air.

'They're all nice …' I said, gesturing towards the men inside.

'But no contenders,' Sam finished my sentence.

We turned away from the dancing bodies inside and looked across the terrace houses tucked into themselves in the dark of our old hometown.

'I think I've realised that even more than a relationship, the one thing I really want is to have a kid,' Sam said. 'If I don't meet someone, I'm going to figure out how to do it on my own.'

I looked at her with envy and wonder. 'What do you mean? Like using a sperm donor?'

Sam blew out a line of smoke. 'Yep.'

'I've thought about it,' I admitted. 'But it seems so hard on your own.'

Sam shrugged. 'I don't know, sometimes I think, do I even want a partner? Is it like a human requirement or cultural conditioning?'

I knew exactly what she meant. I watched a group of women inside who were shouting along to Taylor Swift and shaking and leaping around the kitchen.

Sam passed me the joint. 'And so many male partners don't show up in the same way that the mothers do. I mean, there are partnerships that are more equal. And that's really great for them, but I don't look at them with longing.'

I couldn't shake off my longing though. And I was having my purple patch. There'd been the hot divorcee who liked a drink or ten, and lived in a bunker-like apartment with no windows. His love bombing had fizzled out like a firecracker when things looked like they could actually get serious. There'd been the falling-down-the-rabbit-hole romance with a foreigner I'd met at a wedding who I knew was leaving town. There was the artist with a wicked sense of humour. He had the constitution of a nineteenth-century consumptive – always sniffling in bed with a cold and sleeping with one sock on – afraid of his own shadow or a late-night, romantic walk in the park. And he didn't want children. There was the square-jawed flyer doctor who seemed promising until he fell asleep on our second date while sitting upright in a car on the way to my friend's party. Once there, he flirted with every available warm body and trawled the room trying to score drugs.

So many times, I'd pitched hope against doubt, throwing buckets of optimism at the obvious incompatibilities of the men I was meeting. I'd squinted to look past the red flags waving at me in frenzied semaphore. Everyone had baggage, I told myself. No one was perfect. Surely, he was good enough. Not only that, he had a ready supply of available sperm.

But I was caught in the soul-crushing late-thirties dating dance like so many of my friends. Brilliant and eligible straight, single women, who were doing the limbo, shimmying under a lowering bar of expectations for their relationships with men.

We knew that the men we were dating were not necessarily the making of a lifelong happy match. But it felt like we should overlook that knowledge to get to the destination many of us were hungry for: a family. Should we just concede that while we hadn't found a great love, we'd found someone who could fill enough criteria for the future we hoped for? Even if we suspected that the relationship was sure to implode in the years ahead? Should we – as people had said to Lucie and me – just be less picky?

My friends and I were not just limbo-ing while dating, we were commando crawling at top speed through the mud, muttering encouragement to ourselves and each other: 'No really, I'm fine, he's got some issues but he's great.'

I watched as a man inside at the singles party did a crouching shuffle onto the dance floor, trying to infiltrate the sea of confident women.

In my more generous moments, I saw myself and all these men bobbing in a vast ocean, searching for someone else to keep us afloat. I couldn't dismiss every man as a Peter Pan or a player with the emotional proficiency of a newt (although it felt like newts were the majority). Sure, I'd been rejected, but I'd also felt indifferent towards men who'd pursued me. Although I'd always tried to be polite and upfront when I let them down, I'd no doubt hurt them, in the same way that the men who'd been uninterested in me had hurt me. I'd radiated the same apathy – going on a couple of dates, sometimes even kissing them, taking off our clothes and stepping into each other then politely declining because *I wasn't ready to date* or *I wasn't in the right place* or insert whatever euphemism felt kindest.

When someone didn't want to love you or have a baby with you, it was important to convince yourself that it had nothing to do with you. The timing was wrong. He wasn't willing to commit. He just got divorced. You could always find a friend to corroborate these ideas. Lucie and I could spend hours over a bottle of pinot dissecting his indifference as an *avoidant attachment* style caused by his mother's indifference, his father's absence or the death of his childhood pet ferret.

All my reasoning why it wouldn't work with these men might have been right, but at the end of the night, I was still sleeping alone. I could starfish my limbs across the bed, hogging the covers – which was lovely sometimes, and others, just plain lonely. Some nights I still reached across the bed to find Dave. To hold and be held. Instead, I was jolted by the shock of cold sheets, of nothingness. He was nowhere and I was lost.

The White Rabbit

Two years had passed since I ended my relationship with Dave because I wanted to have children. I was now thirty-nine. All the flings of the last couple of years had sparked out – like the wake of dead stars trailing through the sky.

Unlike other pursuits that you repeated to gain expertise – martial arts, speaking a foreign language, baking sourdough – dating didn't make you win at dating. It didn't bring you any closer to your desired destination: love. The longer I dated, in fact, the further my body travelled from what I hoped would be love's reward: a baby.

So I did what single women in their late thirties do when they're at a loose end: I went to yoga. The studio was draughty and the blow heaters couldn't thaw our feet. I needed a guru and the softly spoken teacher Wendy was ready to fill that vacancy.

'Straighten your arms, tighten your core and reach into the fullness, the realness, the ...' Wendy trailed off. I was waiting. The whole class was waiting. We were reaching for the realness but we were doomed to never find out what lay beyond it. Wendy had a habit of not finishing her sentences.

I glanced at the skinny man on the mat next to me – his feet were pale and flat, like the underbelly of a fish. *Could I love a man with feet like that?*

I remembered the recent blog post I'd worked on with Esther. She'd been giving readers tips on branching out from the internet and embracing chance encounters. 'Go up to a stranger in a café and chat to them,' she said as though it was no big thing. How would I start a conversation with the man next to me?

After class, Wendy drifted around introducing people. 'Ally, this is Pete,' she said, pointing at the skinny man. Finally, Wendy had delivered. My guru had saved me.

Pete was a stooped beanpole with a slight lisp and a boyish face that was lit by a half-smile as though he was always about to make a joke. He eagerly chatted to me as we walked outside to our bikes, which were chained next to each other.

Pete was an accountant and when I told him I was a writer, he was genuinely interested. I pedalled off feeling a sliver of possibility. It's not that I was attracted to him, but I wanted there to be options. I wanted to be wanted.

What I wanted and what I needed were at odds. I needed to face my waning fertility. Since my conversation with Sam, and as the subsequent months of unrewarding dates had passed by, I'd started to seriously consider having a baby alone. I made an appointment with a fertility specialist and did the required blood tests in advance.

The specialist's office was in the same building where my dad had his medical consulting rooms. I didn't want Dad or anyone he worked with to see me there. I didn't want to explain to my family what I was doing. I locked my bike halfway down the block then casually walked past the building, heart galloping, and glanced around. No one there. I turned and quickly ducked inside the sliding doors.

The specialist sat at her desk framed by a bright yellow and orange splashy canvas. She wasn't cold but she wasn't exactly warm. I told her I wanted to have children but I didn't have a partner. I lowered my voice. 'I've been thinking about having a baby, on my own.'

I stared at the doctor, waiting for her reaction. She nodded, unfazed. What had I hoped for? A hand reached across the desk? A sympathetic, *I know, it's such a difficult decision.*

The doctor talked hard facts. 'Your AMH is not bad,' she said. The levels of AMH (anti-mullerian hormone) in my blood were an indication of my ovarian reserve, she explained.

'But AMH is only one part of the picture,' she continued. 'You can't really measure how many years you have left. It doesn't tell us the quality of your remaining eggs.'

I tried not to panic. How many years and eggs did I have left?

She scanned my patient form. 'So how old are you? Right, thirty … nine. Hmm.' This fact seemed to disappoint her. 'You could freeze your eggs but I usually suggest you do that before thirty-eight. After that, the decline in egg quality can be pretty swift. So you don't have much time.'

Time. There it was. For a second, I saw Time as the White Rabbit, littering my youthful eggs as its tail flashed in the distance on the path ahead. I imagined myself chasing along behind the rabbit desperately trying to scoop up my eggs.

I inhaled and held my breath, my chest tight. 'So how does the, um, egg freezing work?'

She launched into a rote monologue, looking slightly bored. 'Well, you'd do self-administered injections of follicle stimulating hormones for about ten to twelve days, the nursing team would talk you through it. You can get bloated. Most people are fine to exercise but some people's ovaries can swell up substantially to about the size of a mango. In which case we'd recommend no exercise so that you don't fall and cause any damage. And then there's a very short procedure under sedation that takes about fifteen minutes where we extract your eggs.'

'How many eggs would you be likely to get at my age?' I swallowed.

She pulled out a graph with bright curving lines and consulted it. 'It's impossible to know exactly but if you were, say under thirty-five ...'

I was no longer under thirty-five.

'We might get between ten to twelve eggs. Which we'd freeze. Then say around eight or nine might survive the thawing process. Then once they're fertilised with sperm, around three might survive. Then there's about a seventy per cent chance of getting pregnant – that's with the under thirty-five-year-old eggs though. If you froze the same number of eggs at the age of forty-four, there's about a seven per cent chance of pregnancy. So the age of the eggs really matters.'

None of this was reassuring.

'Of course, you can also fertilise the eggs and freeze embryos instead but that requires you to choose a sperm donor.'

I felt sick. The specialist closed her folder to wrap things up. 'I think it'd be worthwhile starting fertility counselling. It's mandatory for assisted reproductive treatment and it might help you decide. And there's a solo mums' support group if you're interested in going to that? I can give you the details.' *Interesting*, I thought. *Or sad?* I couldn't decide. There was a tinge of something loser-ish about it, like a twelve-step group for single women desperate for babies.

After the appointment, the patient liaison showed me the numbers for egg freezing. The cycle would be around $4500, the procedure roughly $1200 and then there were the initial storage fees for a year ($500) plus more for ongoing storage costs.

I quickly did the mental calculations and saw the zeroes roll upwards.

I exited and paid the hefty consultation fee, booked a counselling appointment and slunk out onto the busy street, hurriedly putting my helmet on and hopping on my bike to coast down the hill.

As I replayed her advice, I pedalled faster, chasing the White Rabbit into darker, more treacherous thickets. *Time. Decline. Injections. Bloated. Freezing. Sperm. Survive. Costs.* I skidded through orange lights, I swerved around corners. When I arrived at work and fumbled with my bike lock, I was sweating, dizzy. It was all just too much. Too much money. Too much uncertainty. Too much choice. I put two hands on my bike to keep me upright and felt a clench in my gut. I closed my eyes and took some steadying breaths.

At my desk, I stared at the soothing white screen, the blandness of the copywriting work numbed me. I now worked with Sam at an ad agency. She strolled over to my desk, beaming. 'Hey! I've got something to show you.'

It'd been a year since we'd hosted our singles party. Sam leant over my desk and gave me her phone. On her screen was a black-and-white modelling headshot of a twenty-something guy. He had dark, lush wavy curls to his shoulders and olive skin, a perfect mole above his stubbled lips. His gentle brown eyes were staring into the camera intently.

'How hot is he?' she giggled.

The man's name was Artur, a twenty-nine-year-old from the US. 'We video-chatted the other day on FaceTime,' Sam said.

'Wait, so this is the possible sperm donor guy? The nude model?' I asked.

Sam had run a side business in New York – nude-drawing classes for hens' nights featuring young, beautiful, naked male models, and women sitting in front of easels sketching the men and getting drunk on champagne. Sam's old business partner had suggested she contact one of the models, Artur, who was interested in becoming a sperm donor.

Sam couldn't keep the smile from her face. 'I really think he's going to be the future biological father of my child.'

'Hang on, slow down, I need to know exactly what happened,' I said.

Sam laughed. I grabbed a mug from my desk and we ambled to the kitchen to make tea.

While co-workers milled past the kitchen, Sam explained, without any self-consciousness that someone would overhear her.

'I felt like a thirteen-year-old girl calling a boy for the first time on the phone. I was so nervous. I just had no idea what to expect. Like, how do you start a conversation with, "Hey, do you want to give me your genetics?"'

I stayed facing Sam as I flicked the hot water tap. Felt the scalding water rise. Dropped in the tea bag. Slop of milk. Dunk. Dunk. Checked for the right caramel shade to blush through. Took out the bag. Squeezed. Binned. All of it was so automatic that I could keep my eyes on Sam. I didn't want to miss a single expression.

'It all just felt so easy. And he was very straight to the point of like, "Okay, so how do we make this happen?"'

She shook her head in disbelief. 'And then I hung up and just cried. Just like happy, happy tears.' Even as she looked at me now, her eyes were shining.

I held two hands around the mug of tea, like cupping a warm heart. We both stared at Artur's photo on her phone, which sat on the bench in front of us. I felt envious and awestruck. Sam, in her self-possessed Sam-ness had simply made a decision about how to have a baby.

'Maybe he could be your donor too?' Sam struck a comedic pose, shoulders to her ears, both palms pointing skyward.

'Really! Isn't that kind of crazy?' I asked.

'I don't know, is it? I feel like we're just making this up as we go along,' she said.

I turned the idea over – catching her excitement. Maybe the solution was right here.

'I can ask him if he'll speak to you, if you want? He's really lovely.'

Later that day, a message popped up on Facebook from Pete, the tall guy from yoga. He'd bought a play of mine, read it, liked it, and told me how much. *How sweet*, I thought. Then quickly forgot about the interaction.

A few weeks after Sam showed me Artur's photo, I arranged to speak to him. Before I dialled his name, I nervously wrote out some questions which I hid out of view of the screen. What would I say to this complete stranger? Beyond asking about his life and his work and his family, could I ask questions about his health, his sex life, the efficacy and speed of his, um, semen? 'So if you could just rate your sperm on a scale. With *one* being sperm that's about as effective as mayonnaise and *ten* being horse-powered spunk ...'

Definitely not.

While I was worrying, Artur's face appeared on my screen smiling. It was summer in New York, and he was wearing a black singlet so that you could see the muscled cut of his arms. I noticed that a vein ran down his right bicep. His hair was long and wavy, he wore large silver hoop earrings in his ears. He spoke slowly, gently, giving off California vibes; this was a man who woke each day to sunshine.

'So is this the second weirdest phone call you've had, after Sam's?' I asked.

Artur gave a beatific half-smile. 'Yeah, yeah, although, ya know, it wasn't that weird.'

We puttered through some small talk about the difference in seasons between the hemispheres, about how Artur grew up in Texas and his family was from the Dominican Republic. Then I glanced down at my questions and tried to make my voice sound natural. 'So I'm curious, obviously. Why do you want to be a donor, if you don't mind me asking?'

Artur spoke with consideration, stressing each word.

'I've known for a long time that the path that I've chosen in life is challenging for me to do traditional relationships. Uh, so even when it comes to dating, I'm not a monogamous person. I've been in various open, committed things over the years.'

I nodded, trying to reserve my judgement. I thought about one of the men I'd recently dated who'd confessed a few months in that he wasn't really into monogamy. I'd had to restrain myself from letting out a Munch-like scream and ejecting him from my living room. Could I use a sperm donor who had numerous sexual partners at the same time?

I tried to refocus and listen to Artur. 'And then the other thing was I had cousins who struggled to have kids and I saw their struggle ... And I thought it would be nice to have a kid when I was young, younger, and even if I'm not necessarily in their life in a traditional sense, that we could be connected.'

Artur was twenty-nine, close to the age that Dave had been when we broke up. Dave, who at thirty, had been so far from wanting children.

I shook my head in wonder. 'I think it's pretty rare, like, as a twenty-nine-year-old man to want to father a child?'

Artur put his hand on his chest and laughed. 'Well, coming from my community, that's very late.'

I felt myself redden, embarrassed at my rarefied, narrow white view.

'So have you thought about donating through a clinic?' I asked.

He shook his head. 'I don't want to do the anonymous donor thing. Here in New York, I've known some starving artist types or people who were broke who just donate to get paid.'

Unlike in Australia, where it's illegal to be paid for human tissue, meaning that sperm donors are unpaid, the US clinics pay donors. Which is why there are so many more donors in the US, and explains why many egg and sperm donors are young students in need of cash.

'I didn't want to donate to just anyone. That's why Sam and I have been talking about what the kid might go through, what the relationship might look like, what our values are, you know, just lots of things.'

Maybe Artur was judging me too, measuring me to see if I was the right recipient for his sperm. What if I wasn't good enough for him? Maybe I should have changed into something more flattering. I thoughtlessly tugged my t-shirt down a little to reveal some cleavage. But this wasn't a seduction. Or was it?

I looked back at my questions. 'So how do your family feel about you being a donor?' I asked.

Artur let out a 'Ha!'

'My family …' he paused. I waited for a story of struggle, of resisting his family's traditional ideals, as I would have to do if I went down the path of solo motherhood.

'My family,' he repeated, 'is so supportive of everything that I do.'

I sat back, absorbing this. I envied his family's lack of judgement. 'That's great, I wish my parents were like that.'

Artur waited for me to go on, head cocked to the side.

I took a deep confessional breath. 'I'm still, like, considering this solo mum thing. I'm not really sure where I'm at with it. I'm not quite where Sam is. I haven't made my mind up yet.' Artur looked at me with kind eyes.

After we hung up, I exhaled. Artur was a good person. But I didn't feel the same spark that Sam had felt. I couldn't help picturing Artur in my life and asking the questions that came with that image. Could I love him? Could I sleep with him? Could he father my child? No matter how sterile the biological process of artificial insemination was, it was almost impossible for me to separate it from desire. I liked Artur, he was handsome and kind, but his earnest sensibility was at odds with my pragmatic, neurotic self. He just wasn't my type.

Also, I wondered whether sharing a donor with Sam would be a mistake. Our friendship was harmonious. But what if one of us had trouble conceiving? What grief and conflict might lie ahead of us? What if we both conceived and then had children who were siblings? Our friendship would stretch into something else, something binding and familial. How would our different parenting styles clash and cause conflict and envy for our future siblings? If Sam and I had a shared donor, we would be wedded together for a life that was, at its best, miraculous and love-filled, at worst, heavy with obligation and resentment.

Sam was also sure about her chosen path and I was not. Maybe Sam was better adjusted, more progressive and adventurous than I was. She had a big loving family who had embraced her chutzpah, while I was still wrestling with my mother's doubts.

I often heard those doubts in my head, the echo of her words, 'Children need a mother and a father.' I didn't agree with my mother, at least not intellectually. But her view was lodged like a boulder between me and choosing to become a solo parent. I couldn't see a way around it.

❦

Years ago, after my grandfather, my mother's remaining parent, had died, my family exited the beige funeral home and walked to the car. My mum turned to my brothers and me and said, 'I'm an orphan now.'

Her voice caught in a way that I'd never heard, revealing a gully of sadness rushing beneath.

'Oh, Mum,' I said.

'The only thing I have to look forward to is having grandchildren,' she said, her voice transitioning to self-pity.

My brothers and I groaned loudly and exclaimed over each other.

'Oh God!'

'Mum!'

'Seriously?'

It wasn't the first time she'd said this to us. My brothers and I laughed together as we got into the car.

My mum's lament about grandchildren was annoying, in the way that any mother's lament is, but I didn't begrudge her that hope. I wanted to have children; I understood her longing. But how could I meet my mother's hopes while going against her strongly held beliefs?

Even though I'd lived overseas for ten years, even though I'd made an unconventional career as a writer, even though I'd had a free and independent life, was I really going to do something that my own flesh and blood disapproved of? Especially when it came to something as fundamental as making my own family, for which I would need my family's support more than anything.

Perhaps underneath my so-called bravery and independence, I was lily-livered and obedient – a child seeking my parents' approval. Or maybe I was too hung up on love, on the addictive possibility of new romance. Unable to let go of the hope that maybe I'd still meet someone, so I could fall in line and have a conventional family and leave these complicated questions behind.

Zygote

After the usual banalities of an online flirtation where we humbly bragged about our accomplishments and shared crumbs of vulnerabilities to make us look more attractive, Pete asked if I wanted to go to a movie.

As I walked to the date, I quelled my nerves by repeating in my mind: *You're just meeting another zygote.* Something about picturing a man as a tiny cluster of cells in his mother's womb, pre-embryo, always relaxed me.

When I got to the cinema, I looked down from the balcony to the bustle of the food court. Pete was sitting at a table, his large frame bent over his phone. There was something endearing about him sitting there. He was on time (tick). He didn't have a drink yet which meant he was waiting for me to arrive to order one (tick). He looked slightly nervous which meant he cared (tick). It was these small things that made an outsized difference in matters of courting.

When Pete saw me, he jumped up and opened his giant arms, enclosing me in an enthusiastic hug. He said my name loudly, as though we were being reunited after a long trip.

'I've bought the movie tickets but I haven't got any drinks yet. Do you want a drink? They have a bar. I need a drink.' He was talking fast and gesturing with his long arms.

'Um, yeah, I can get the drinks,' I said. 'So that we're being equitable or whatever?'

'Of course, I want to empower you to be equitable. You buying me a drink doesn't emasculate me at all,' he deadpanned.

I laughed. He had a way of twisting his neuroses into self-deprecating charm.

After the movie, we talked without pause. The date was a chorus of *so do I's!*

Each similarity that we discovered was a revelation, as though our vegetarianism, love of tea and our mutual agreement on the merits of various films from our teenagehood was a sign of being fated.

After the movie and a passionate dissection of it over dinner, we ended up at Heartbreaker, an American-style dive bar in the city. It was a late-night place with neon signs on the walls, a pool table and a jukebox. There was plenty of room, but we crammed ourselves into the corner of a booth and probed each other's pasts and quirks to try to figure out whether we could fall in love.

'I've definitely got a bit of George Costanza in me,' he admitted.

I leant towards him to be heard over the music. 'Well, you're not bald, at least.'

'No, at least I don't have to be neurotic about being bald, I can just be neurotic about being neurotic,' he said.

I widened my eyes at him, trying to decide how I felt about this.

'Neurotic about what?' I asked. I felt like a detective searching for clues.

'Most things, it takes me a while to get comfortable in a relationship,' his eyes jumped around the room.

'I think most people are like that.' I was easily won over by this admission.

'Yeah, I suppose, I think it's a confidence thing,' said Pete. 'Like what you've done, become a writer. I always wanted to do something like that but I didn't really have the balls. I'm better at being a lovable failure.'

There was a radical honesty and wryness to his words that made him more likable than loser-ish. 'That's why I tend to fall for women who are smarter and more ambitious and more successful than I am.'

He looked at me meaningfully. I knew he'd said this to other women in other corner booths in other bars in the past. I didn't mind.

'Like you,' he said.

'Thank you.' My eyes skittered around the room. I didn't know how to arrange my face, I felt so intently looked at.

'Would it be too forward if I kissed you?' he asked.

It was the same every time, the pre-kiss teenage nerves, my desire to flee. I tried to feign cool.

'It would be forward, but not too forward.'

Pete leant over and kissed me.

The neon signs didn't flicker; the room didn't go quiet but it was nice to be kissed, to be wanted.

Over the next few months, Pete and I fell into an amiable togetherness. We rode our bikes to shows and lay in parks reading the Saturday newspaper, we debated the merit of books and movies and TV shows. He was always willing to drive me places and make me eggs in the morning. He was the father to a young boy, a five-year-old, from a previous partnership. This didn't scare me; it endeared me to him more. I told him I was looking for a committed relationship; that I wanted to have children. 'I'd like to have at least five siblings for my son,' Pete said as I lay on his chest in bed. I looked up at him. 'Kidding. Just one. Maybe two. Or three.' He wiggled his eyebrows up and down and made me laugh.

❦

I was waiting in the empty foyer of a terrace house in a suburb just east of the city filled with doctors' offices. I heard the creak of the stairs as the fertility counsellor descended.

My whereabouts was a secret. Because how did you tell someone in the early days of a relationship that you'd been considering having a baby alone? My unfolding relationship was not at pace with this kind of revelation. It was one thing to tell Pete I wanted to have a family. It was another to tell him how far I'd be willing to go to have one. Revealing this, I secretly felt, would dull the shine of my attractiveness. It would expose me as a desperate, single woman; a woman who couldn't find a man to have a baby with her.

Upstairs, in a small room with anodyne cream and yellow furniture, I sat opposite the counsellor, whose long straw-coloured hair blended with the backdrop.

She smiled at me. She waited.

'So I'm not really clear if this appointment is to assess my sanity or whether it's for me to figure out whether I could become a mother on my own?' I asked.

'It's for you.' She smiled but kept her mouth closed.

We were here, she reassured me, so that I could ask questions, and talk about any of my concerns. We were also here because counselling is required by law in Victoria according to the *Assisted Reproductive Treatment Act.*

'I'm still trying to make a decision about having a baby on my own. I've started seeing this guy, and it's going well, but I'm thirty-nine and I can't really predict …'

I trailed off, because the entire predicament of being a woman dating in your late thirties who wanted children filled up that silence.

I was in an impossible situation. I was measuring love's potential against an unseen process of decay inside my own body. How many eggs was I willing to sacrifice to see if love panned out? Was this potential relationship worth three months of eggs? Six? Could I give up half-a-dozen eggs plus a calcifying womb to see if love worked out? How long could I let the waiting eggs inside me age before they crumbled into cakey mothballs? And even if love did work out, how soon was not too insane to make a baby with a new partner? Next year? Next month? Next Tuesday?

My romantic life was out of sync with my reproductive timeline. Each of my dates had an invisible pressure hovering over them. My budding relationship felt like it needed to be accelerated towards a false intimacy.

As I explained all this as best as I could, the counsellor radiated understanding. Her empathy made me want to scream, to pitch furniture upside down and send objects soaring at the window to smash through the glass. *Don't you see*, I wanted to yell. *Don't you get how impossible this all is?*

'Given this new relationship,' she said slowly, 'I suggest you freeze your eggs, then you'll give yourself some options.' She shifted in her seat as though the problem was solved, our time was up. But I didn't have the money to freeze my eggs. Even if I did, I remembered the diminishing returns the specialist had described for women freezing their eggs over the age of thirty-eight. I knew that it was a wonky insurance policy for a future pregnancy.

The counsellor was on the side of the world and the world wanted to believe that love and romance would always win. I wanted to believe it too.

As I left the appointment, I made a mental pros and cons list about Pete. There were so many good things about him. He was kind. He was funny. He was unfailingly encouraging about my work. A few nights earlier, as we walked through the Exhibition Gardens near the city, the dark elms looming above us, I worried aloud about my tenuous financial existence as a freelancer.

'Maybe I just go full-time with the copywriting. Like give up my own writing and get a real job.'

'Don't do it. Don't get a full-time job. You're too talented. Keep writing,' Pete said it without a beat, without any doubt. I felt buoyed and protected by his conviction.

But there was also the neurotic side of Pete that drove me to distraction. The side that constantly complained about his ex-partner in a way that made me suspect there hadn't been enough time since the end of that relationship and ours. The side that called and texted me all day, every day in a way that I found cloying. Only a week ago, I'd asked him to ease up on talking about his ex and give me a few days of breathing space. I had deadlines for a musical I was writing. I needed to be able to think. That evening, as I rode my bike home from work, I heard my phone bleating.

I veered off into a laneway and pulled my phone out of my bag. Pete's grinning photo flashed on-screen. I thought about not answering but I knew he'd just call again. I got off my bike and unclicked my helmet so I could wedge my phone to my ear.

'Hey, what's up?' I sounded cold but I didn't care.

'Hey!' Pete was jaunty. 'I know you said this morning you didn't want me to call but I just wanted to say sorry for calling so much.'

'Right, okay, this is kind of ridiculous, Pete.'

'I know but … it's nice to hear your voice.' I could hear his cheeky, wheedling grin.

I couldn't help laughing. 'I'm gonna go. I'm riding home.'

'Okay, talk to you tomorrow, babe. Or not, I mean, talk to you in a few days. Good luck with your writing. Your musical is going to be incredible!'

I hung up and sighed. I clicked my helmet back on.

Pete was a great friend, but maybe that was all he should be: a friend. It wasn't only his cloying nature that was giving me pause. The attraction that I thought would develop hadn't sparked. Perhaps my inability to feel desire was evidence that I was incapable of really, truly committing to the real deal when it presented itself. Maybe I was just overlooking all the good things about Pete as an act of self-sabotage? Everyone had flaws.

There was another terrible truth lurking that did nothing to save me from my present or even, possibly, my future. I needed to make a decision about the baby thing. Time, that White Rabbit, was disappearing around a corner with my basket of eggs. I slung my leg over my bike, as the rain began. I pedalled hard, all the way home, hoping to catch him before he disappeared.

Shitty Options

Not everyone was waiting for love to arrive so they could have a baby.

One early summer weekend, my friends and I jammed into a car to head down to the coast. Sam was behind the wheel and her car was filled with dogs and bags; Salt 'n' Pepa played through the speakers. In the back seat, crammed between us all was Artur. Sam had flown her sperm donor over from New York. When I saw him, he greeted me affectionately, without blinking, even though last time we'd spoken I'd been considering him as a donor.

We sang along loudly to the music. 'I'm hungry, are we there yet? I need snacks,' I called from the back seat.

Sam laughed. 'You're such a baby. You're always hungry. You can't even survive for half an hour without a snack.'

'I have low blood sugar!' I protested, which was entirely made up.

At the beach house the next morning, as my friends bustled around the kitchen and I emptied the dishwasher, Sam appeared and handed Artur what looked like a small plastic cup. It was a medical specimen jar. Everyone stopped their movement and clatter. We stared at Artur. We were witnessing what could be a life-making transaction. There was silence. Then. 'Is there internet here?' Artur asked in his laidback drawl. We all tried to stay straight-faced. Artur dutifully disappeared into the bedroom, returning a little later with the cup filled with sperm. Sam went into her bedroom to inseminate herself with a needleless syringe. Now all she had to do was wait.

That afternoon, Sam and I sat on our towels on the beach watching Artur in the distance. He stood with his legs in a V-shape, feet digging into the sand, gazing at the sea. Here was a man who was unafraid to fly ten thousand miles across the world to give a woman he barely knew a baby. Sure, he got an Australian trip out of it, and a legal contract had been drawn up to protect both he and Sam, but Artur was genuine. He was doing this for the right reasons. 'I know I'm not here for a holiday,' he had said to Sam.

'So, would you sleep with him?' I asked as we looked on at Artur's smooth, lean body on the shoreline. We giggled. 'Sure,' Sam said, 'if it wasn't going to fuck things up.'

We watched Artur towel the long, wet tendrils of his hair.

'We're going to talk more later about what our plans are for the future if I get pregnant. I just can't get over it. He's everything I could have asked for,' Sam said.

Later, as the sun sank closer to the horizon, after I'd washed off the salt and sand in the outdoor shower, I passed Artur and Sam sitting on the back porch. They both had tears in their eyes but it wasn't sadness I was witnessing. Artur leant over and hugged Sam and I could hear them talking in low voices. I went up to my bedroom and lay on the bed and returned Pete's third missed call.

'How's it going at the beach?' he asked.

I picked at the edge of a fringed cushion with my fingernail as I painted a picture of sun and surf and friends. I omitted the real story about Sam and her donor. If I spoke it aloud, something in my voice might betray that I wanted a child so badly that I'd considered doing it on my own too.

Later that week, I met Lucie for dinner at a packed vegetarian restaurant wedged between record stores and cafés on an eclectic strip in the city's north.

'So, how's Pete? Do you like him yet?' Lucie grinned.

I shovelled in a mouthful of noodles and chewed to avoid answering. Finally, I swallowed.

'He's fine. He's lovely but, you know, I'm ...' I shrugged.

'Mm, yeah. You've been saying that for a while.'

'I know but it's not as easy as just breaking up with him.'

Lucie nodded.

'I'm thirty-nine and he's lovely on paper, like a great partner ...'

Lucie made a 'mmm' sound as she ate her noodles. She understood.

'And he's got some issues with ...' I dropped my voice, 'getting it up.'

A small smile lit Lucie's face.

'And, like, if we have a baby together, how is he going to *deliver*?'

'Yeah that's hard ... that he's not ... hard,' Lucie said.

I inhaled a sip of my wine and started coughing. 'Stop it,' I said, trying not to laugh.

I groaned. 'I can't figure out if I should just, like, end it and have a baby on my own.'

'Ughhh,' Lucie screwed her face up in thought. 'It's tricky when you have to choose between two shitty options.' This was the thing I loved about Lucie, her unfiltered honesty. Right now, it was the thing I most hated.

'I don't see them as shitty options.' I was trying to keep the fury out of my voice.

'Yeah, sure, I just mean, you know,' Lucie backpedalled in a way that was trying for convincing.

Shitty options. Solo motherhood would be bloody hard. Sure. But Lucie was implying that choosing to mother alone would be like waving a flag of defeat in the air. *She couldn't find a man to love her*, the mean girls in my mind snickered. *Not enough to give her a baby*. She believed, and maybe I did too, that this choice would brand me as single for eternity.

Medical History

As a child, I was a believer in romance. Sitting in the back seat of the car, I begged my mum to tell me the story of my parents' engagement in the late 1970s.

'Dad was planning to go overseas to study. So it was either get married or break up,' Mum recounted. 'So we got married.'

This was not what I wanted to hear. Surely there must have been something more: a moonlit walk, a ring in a cigarette packet, a bended knee outside the hospital after their night shift. 'But who proposed?' I asked. I knew this story well but each time I demanded another crumb of detail.

My parents glanced at each other in the front seat, a look forming between them that was killing me. I had to know.

'I think I proposed,' Mum said.

'No, no one did any proposing.' Dad pulled a zipping manoeuvre to get into the left lane and darted through the traffic lights before they turned red.

'Neil!' Mum said. 'Was that really necessary? Slow down.'

'Who *proposed*?' I pressed forward against my seatbelt.

Mum shook her head slightly to indicate that she was either disappointed with my dad, disappointed with my questions or disappointed with the past. 'No one. There was no proposal, we just agreed.'

Just over a year after they were married, at the age of twenty-eight, my mum fell pregnant. There had been no discussion, no formal decision, it had just happened. 'We were both very excited,' Mum smiled.

In July 1979 at the Royal Women's Hospital in Melbourne – just across from the university where my parents had first met while studying medicine – I was yanked into the world with cold metal forceps.

This story of my parents' marriage and my own creation dovetailed with another story – a thorny and sometimes ugly story – of donor conception in Australia.

Almost a year after I was born, in that very same hospital, in June 1980, another baby girl was born: Australia's first IVF baby, Candice Reed, who emerged, obsidian newborn eyes blinking into the lights of the *60 Minutes* camera crew positioned to document the 'test tube' miracle. To the public, the idea of extracting an egg from a woman's body must have seemed futuristic and outlandish. Not to mention, adding sperm to that egg in a dish, then placing a living thing back into a woman's body to grow a baby.

Alongside donor insemination, IVF treatment became more available at fertility clinics over the next ten years, but only for married couples. Single women and lesbian couples were denied assisted reproductive treatment by law in some states and clinic policy in others.

Running parallel to the medical establishment, lesbians had long been the pioneers of donor insemination. In the early '80s lesbians had started forming self-insemination networks in cities across Australia. There was a risk though. Getting a partner or friend to artificially inseminate you outside of a clinic was a criminal offence.

When I found this out, I was shocked. What else didn't I know? I needed the full story. I casually mentioned to my dad that I was doing some research about the history of IVF in Victoria. 'Just for something I'm writing,' I mumbled.

Dad knew everyone medical in Melbourne. He puffed up his chest in a way that suggested he had a lead. 'You need to talk to John McBain, he's an IVF specialist. I know him from uni. He was part of that team that made the first IVF baby here.'

A few weeks later, I watched McBain's face appear on-screen, in front of a photo backdrop of amber leaves and his farmhouse. 'Let me start at the beginning,' McBain began in his Scottish brogue, as though we were entering the land of fairy tales. And in some ways, it felt like we were stepping into a weird past where trolls guarded bridges and, on the other side, beautiful children skipped out of reach of their would-be mothers.

In the late 1990s, McBain kept meeting women who were hungry to have children. In his clinic at Melbourne IVF, more and more single women and same-sex couples were making appointments. McBain explained the laws at the time that restricted IVF treatment. 'Had I decided to do anything, to experiment on an embryo, to observe it even, that would have led to my program being closed down and me being at risk of four years jail. There was a similar penalty for treating women who were unmarried.'

I pictured one of these women, after her appointment, sitting quietly behind her steering wheel, so filled with a ravening want only to be told *no*; wanting to smash the windscreen with her bare fists.

At the time, DIY home insemination was often a single woman's only option. For many lesbian couples, donor conception outside of the medical realm allowed agency and freedom from the male-dominated fertility industry. McBain believed the use of fresh, unscreened sperm was risky. 'I thought this was a public health matter,' he told me. 'So, through ultimate frustration I decided the best way was to sue the Victorian government in the Federal Court.'

McBain took action in the Federal Court, challenging the laws that restricted 'socially infertile' women – those who were single or in same-sex couples – from having babies through assisted medical means. First, he had to find a respondent – a single woman who would agree to go public for the case. It wasn't easy. After asking roughly fifteen women, finally Leesa Meldrum, a single woman who wanted to conceive on her own, agreed. They eventually went to the High Court where McBain argued that the Victorian laws conflicted with federal sex-discrimination legislation.

The night before the case, McBain was at home when the landline rung. It was the late Catholic bioethicist Nicholas Tonti-Filippini on the line. He pleaded with McBain not to go ahead with the case – arguing that it was going to destroy the whole concept of the fabric of the family. McBain was unswayed.

They won the case, much to the dismay of the Catholic Church. Outside the court, speaking to reporters, Cardinal George Pell said, 'We are on the verge of creating a whole new generation of stolen children.'

The question of who has the right be a parent has always been fraught in Australia. There is the long and traumatic history of removing children from Aboriginal families that continues on from the Stolen Generation in the form of 'child protection'. Pell was equating the identity-shattering pain inflicted on Aboriginal children taken from their families with what donor-conceived children raised by one or two mums would feel.

The McBain ruling was controversial across church and state and the public. It caused a schism in the Labor party and drew criticism from conservatives. Liberal Prime Minister John Howard said, 'We do take the view that, all things being equal, children are entitled to the opportunity of both a mother and a father.'

'It threw the government into a bit of a spin,' McBain explained. 'They said, okay, you've won that but they'll have to be medically infertile before you're allowed to treat them.' So with a clever interpretation, the law was restricted to women who were medically infertile.

I imagined myself as a woman in her late thirties walking into an IVF clinic in the 2000s, just twenty or so years ago. I would have had to come prepared with a lie about 'trying' naturally for more than a year to prove I was medically infertile. This was, obviously, difficult to do if you were single or in a same-sex relationship.

Inspired by the image of Leesa Meldrum on the front page of the paper, Leanne Haynes became one of the first solo mothers in Victoria. Now a former schoolteacher in her fifties, Leanne agreed to talk to me about what it was like being on the vanguard of women doing it alone. In the background of our call, I could hear her donor-conceived eight-year-old son and thirteen-year-old daughter bickering. She told them off, heaved a sigh then came back on the line. She explained to me how she became one of many Melbourne women who were fertility fugitives, travelling across state lines to be artificially inseminated in Sydney in the early 2000s.

'I knew the Virgin Blue timetable off by heart.' She laughed. In the morning, she would pee on a stick to see if she was ovulating and then hop on a plane to Sydney – sometimes making the round-trip in one day to be back in the classroom teaching by the afternoon. Haynes travelled across state lines to Bondi ten failed times in 2002 to try to have a baby until she was finally deemed 'medically infertile'. Only then, in 2003, was she finally able to access IVF treatment in Victoria. After years of insemination, and failed IVF attempts, Haynes' daughter was born after her fifteenth embryo transfer in 2006. 'I didn't know what happiness was until I held her,' she said. 'That was when I felt truly happy. You can't put a value on that.'

Despite the shift in the law, there was still a stigma in the early 2000s around becoming a mother without a man in the picture. What if men – gasp! – were done away with altogether? Spurred in part by the controversy of McBain's successful case, in 2002, the Victorian Law Reform Commission held an inquiry into the laws governing assisted reproductive technology and adoption.

Over the following years, gay and lesbian activists used the commission as a platform to campaign for equal status for same-sex relationships under the law, and for single women and same-sex couples to be able to access assisted reproductive treatment without being discriminated against. The Fertility Access Rights Lobby (which later became the Rainbow Families

Council) formed a revolutionary campaign called 'Love Makes a Family' in 2004.

The campaign was persistent and inspired. They sent photos of their families to politicians; they organised media training for gay and lesbian families; they wrote letters; they met with MPs; they sat with their babies in the public gallery of Parliament when the Assisted Reproductive Treatment (ART) bill was being debated. They gathered with prams and grandparents on the steps of Parliament. They argued that women should have autonomy over their reproductive rights.

The campaign's goal was to change people's hearts and minds by sharing personal stories and forming bonds and connections with others to illuminate a shared humanity, no matter a person's gender, sexuality or relationship status. And in doing so, transform the law.

Finally, in 2010, as a result of the inquiry and the tireless campaigning of gay and lesbian activists, the law changed in a number of ways to recognise same-sex families and to lift the medical infertility barrier in Victoria. This meant that women in Victoria no longer had to prove they were medically infertile to access reproductive treatment (although it's still a barrier to accessing Medicare rebates for treatment). Police and child protection order checks were introduced at the same time for parents-to-be, coinciding with same-sex couples and single women now having access to assisted reproduction.

I asked McBain what these checks were about. 'It was the same group of people, the Catholic hierarchy, influencing the Catholic cabinet ministers, who got the police checks brought in because they didn't want lesbians having children so they could abuse them. Just imagine the irony of the Catholic Church saying that.' McBain all but rolled his eyes. The police checks were abolished in 2020.

It was only in 2017, when the restrictions that women had to prove their medical infertility to access ART were lifted in South Australia that it finally became legal, across Australia, for single women and same-sex couples to use donor sperm.

There was no legal obstacle to my getting pregnant alone through an IVF clinic so why was I still struggling to make the decision?

These laws and regulations were written to protect future children. But from what? Was a fatherless existence so terrible? If I conceded that my future child could have negative feelings about the absence of a second parent – especially when faced with the majority of other families – was this a reason *not* to have a child at all? Many fathers failed their children. Wasn't no father better than a deadbeat dad? Or was I letting my blind hunger for a baby get in the way of reason and damning a child to an unhappy life? Was I being *selfish*, the word my mum had used to describe solo mothers.

I couldn't ask my mother what she meant by those words because I was afraid to touch something so personal and fraught between us. But there was another story. A clue perhaps. In 1978, my aunt, my father's unmarried sister, became pregnant. Was it a one-night stand? A brief romance? No one knew or dared ask, but recently my aunt told me that at the time, she was turning thirty and thinking about having a child. Her baby was due to be born one month after I would arrive. Concerned about her family's reaction and not wanting to upstage my married parents who were producing the longed-for grandchild, my aunt had kept it a secret. But at six months pregnant, it was hard to hide. Her mother confronted her. Her father never once spoke of it. My aunt's pregnancy, it seemed, had brought my grandparents shame. But it also brought them a beloved grandson – my cousin – who was raised as the son of a single mother.

Shame. Is that what my motherhood as a single woman conjured for my own parents? That musty smell that still clung to a single, pregnant woman?

Shame. That controlling force. It poured down from the rule-makers, the state, the church, and made its way like tap water into the homes and lives and minds of the people. Shame, which decreed that there was one, narrow path in life and that we must all adhere to it.

If I dug down, layer upon layer, like a dog scrabbling in the dirt for a bone, was that what I would find underneath all this: the desiccated husk of shame? A shame that dictated to me: you must fall into line. You must marry a boy – any boy, but preferably one who doesn't deviate from the norm himself. You must couple with someone whose life fits in neat and sensible rows. Straight. Financially secure. Steady. Only then can you have children.

I had found myself that kind of man in Dave – albeit one who was a creative type and an American (two strikes) but in every other way fitted the conventional requirements. The problem was, he hadn't wanted to do the most conventional of things: make a family.

McBain had seen the same things in his IVF clinic. 'One of the most distressing circumstances we see is where a man says, "I'm not ready, not quite ready, not ready yet."'

I squirmed in my seat. 'That was definitely the case for me with my ex-boyfriend … I had to get out.'

He nodded, sympathetic. 'It's a foolish man who stands in the way of a woman wanting to have a child.'

I felt a wash of bitter triumph. He continued, 'If you're in a relationship and the woman wants to have a child and you see this as an ongoing relationship, then I think it's cruel and selfish for the man not to agree to that.'

I'd been vindicated but it didn't matter, it was too late for regret. I needed to move forward from the past.

It was almost four decades since my mother had given birth to me – such a short span in the vastness of history, and yet my generation had moved to a different planet. We lived in a universe where people fell in love through the invisible portal of the internet, where same-sex couples could get married. Where, I, as a single woman, no longer needed romance because I could make a child by walking into an IVF clinic.

Choice

A few weeks after our beach trip to get Sam pregnant, I got on Facebook. In the search bar, I typed the name of a group that I'd heard about: Australia Solo Mothers by Choice. The group was private but I checked and re-checked my settings. I imagined nightmarish scenarios where I'd post a comment – *I'm thirty-nine and my last good eggs are suiciding. Help! Send sperm!* – that would appear to my entire friend feed, including Pete.

After my request was approved, I lurked among the then 1400-strong vocal chorus of women and observed. The group was started by Melbourne solo mum Michelle Galea in 2013, with just a few hundred women, initially for friends, and friends of friends. It now had a long waitlist of member requests pending and, by 2023, the number would balloon to more than 2800. Posts were peppered with acronyms I'd never heard of and read something like this:

Hey! I'm ttc [trying to conceive] my second child. My family were really supportive about me ttc my first one but they don't think I should have another baby. For those with more than one, do you have any regrets?

My test was negative. Again. My period arrived just as I was going into a meeting at work. How does everyone else deal with this stuff?

My boy is almost three and he's starting to ask questions about why he doesn't have a daddy. Wondering how other solo mamas have dealt with this?

The group was a disparate community united by a shared desire. There were women dipping their toes into the pond of assisted conception to find answers, others who were going through arduous rounds of embryo transfers, pregnant mothers and many who were already solo parents. The wall was populated with questions about everything from balance bikes to bassinets and blastocysts (embryos at around day five of conception).

The community was started as a place to organise in-person gatherings but it had grown to provide support, information, personal anecdotes, birth announcements and empowering memes. It was where women grieved, celebrated, vented and escaped the judgement of a world that had not entirely caught up to the unconventional path of solo motherhood.

I marvelled at all these women who had already wrestled with and made this choice. I, on the other hand, still couldn't decide. Mostly, I couldn't decide what to do about Pete.

'The sexual chemistry between us is incredible,' Pete had said that morning as we sat in his sunlit garden under a lemon-scented gum tree, eating gluten-free pancakes that he'd lovingly made.

'It is good,' I murmured in as convincing a voice as I could muster.

'Incredible,' he deadpanned.

His small jokes disarmed and charmed me, and made me think, *I should try to make this work*.

Pete could sense something was off between us though. He was constantly 'checking in' with me and asking why I was so distant. Not ten minutes after I'd left his house, he'd written me a text message: *Hey, is everything okay?* I was irritated by the message. I was irritated that he wanted to give me a key to his house. I was irritated that he wanted to introduce me to his son so early in our relationship. All these eager offers, if I'd loved him, if I'd desired him, would normally have thrilled me, but instead I felt trapped.

I went to Sydney for a few days for some work meetings and stayed with my brother Nick. Sitting in his back garden, as we drank beers in the subtropical shimmer of a Sydney afternoon, I explained the dilemma about Pete. My brother has a sage and contemplative way of listening. 'You can't just string him along. He doesn't seem to be making you happy, either,' he said.

'I just keep hoping it's going to work out, somehow magically. And dating again, trying to meet someone new ... ugh.'

My brother took a slug of beer.

'You can't stay with him because you don't want to be single.'

'I know but I really want to have a baby.'

'Do you want to have a baby with him, though?' Nick scrunched his face up.

I sighed. 'No, not really.'

Nick was right. I wanted to have a baby so badly that I was trying to bend the nearest available man into the shape of someone I could love.

When I got back to Melbourne, Pete picked me up from the airport and drove me to my writer's studio, which was in a converted 1800s convent. I sat at my desk as far as possible from where he was perched opposite me on the two-seater couch. As I looked at him, I felt a wave of affection and pity and revulsion rise up in me.

'You're really great,' I said, in not the most original way to preface a break-up, 'but I just don't feel like this is working.'

Pete's face turned ashen. He slowly rocked his head and shoulders forward and back in tiny increments then finally spoke. 'Yeah, I figured as much. I mean, you've been kind of weirdly distant.'

'I know, I'm sorry, I was just trying to figure out how I felt.'

'I really like you, Ally.' He fixed his gaze steadily on me. His eyes were limpid, like a Labrador begging for food. It was excruciating.

'I know, I like you too,' I said. It was true. 'I just feel like maybe we should be friends, not partners.'

Pete winced. 'Right, okay. I mean I thought we were more than friends but …'

There was a terrible silence.

'I really do think you're terrific,' I said. *Terrific? Why was I talking like I was a gal in a 1940s movie?*

'Well, I'm obviously not that *terrific* or you'd want to stay with me,' Pete said.

'I'm sorry … But I really hope you meet someone. Which you will.'

'Stop being so magnanimous.' He tried to curl his lips into a smile. 'You're supposed to be upset.'

After he left, I sat on the couch and sobbed. I sobbed so hard and loud that I worried my sobs were echoing through the quiet hallway into the neighbouring writers' studios. I imagined the other writers stopping, pens poised, ears pricking, as they jotted me down: *Through the walls, a woman weeps.* I didn't want to be a character in a story.

I pressed Nick's number on my phone. He answered straight away from Sydney – he was probably standing in one of the lush, wealthy gardens he worked in, dirt under his fingernails.

I somehow got out the words through choking sobs.

'I'm sorry.' The kindness in his voice tipped me over the edge. I was crying harder than before.

'I really want to have a baby. I'm worried it's going to be too late.'

'Yeah, I know.' He didn't try to console me with false promises that everything would be okay.

'If I have a baby on my own, will you move back to Melbourne?'

'I promise you,' he paused for emphasis, 'that if you have a baby on your own, I'll move to Melbourne.' His certainty made me start crying again.

'I'm afraid of doing it alone.'

'I know.'

Over the next week, I let myself wallow but, as the days passed, my sadness evaporated like haze on the horizon. I realised I was grieving my future family, not the loss of a man.

I called Sam a few days later. She answered, groggy, even though it was the afternoon.

'Did I wake you up?'

'I've been sleeping a lot lately. I'm pregnant.'

I let out a cry of excitement. I thought I would feel envious but I was thrilled. Sam had wanted this so badly. She deserved it.

After our wonder had subsided, she asked, 'What's happening with you?'

'Well ... I ended it with Pete. Which sucks, but it's also a relief. I mean, this is kind of awful but I don't really feel sad about not being with him, just sad that I don't have someone to have a baby with.'

'Oh yeah ... I remember feeling like that. But, you know, once I let the sadness out, it made way for all these new narratives I hadn't even considered.'

Hearing her words, that's when I knew.

My romantic future could wait, but the cold, hard biological facts meant that having a baby could not. There was another narrative: a story of being done with waiting, a story of agency, a story of my own making.

Ready

One September morning in 2018, without telling a soul where I was going, I rode my bike through the drizzle, up a church-spired hill in the inner city. I finally crested the hill, panting and frazzled, both sweaty and cold, and locked up my bike.

The church hall was draughty – filled with the kind of chill that Melbourne spring had perfected. In a wonky circle sat a group of about twenty women. The blonde facilitator smiled at me kindly as I took an empty seat. Down one end of the circle were women with babies and toddlers, their offspring obliviously babbling and squalling. At the other end were the rest of us – the single women who were considering having a baby or were trying to conceive. The meeting, a support group for solo mothers by choice, was run by the Victorian Assisted Reproductive Treatment Authority (VARTA). I felt like an imposter, a tourist. What was I even doing here?

The meeting topic was, ironically, dating. The conversation tentatively pinged around the circle. No one talked about a longing for romance, for love, for partnership. Many of the women with children said they didn't have the time or inclination to date: their lives were busy and rewarding, and they were only interested in a partner who could add something to their family.

A brunette with a wry sense of humour who I decided could be a future friend was telling a story that was the inverse of a romantic narrative. Her name was Mara and she had a six-month-old baby girl, Rose, who had Mara's startling blue eyes. When Mara started IVF, it had coincided with the start of a new relationship. 'He was on board with what I was doing but I couldn't figure out how to let the relationship unfold naturally while I tried to get pregnant artificially,' she shrugged. The relationship had petered out as Mara went through round upon round of treatment until she eventually got pregnant.

Another mother in the circle laughingly confessed, 'I used to date for sperm.' The phrase chimed in my head with a ding of recognition. She was, essentially, looking for a man to have a baby with but she realised it was an impossible pressure to put on her romantic life.

One woman with a toddler told us how she'd recently met her girlfriend. She'd made the decision to be a solo mum at twenty-five. 'All I wanted was to be a mum and I knew that being gay, one day I'd have to have a donor,' she said. When she went to a fertility clinic though, she encountered opposition. They made her apply to the board of the clinic to be approved for fertility treatment because, they said, she was too young to know her mind. 'They made me write a letter,' she told us with fury in her voice.

The clinic had granted her permission, which led to two unsuccessful rounds of treatment. In the end, she had fallen pregnant through home insemination, using donor sperm from a friend.

After she finished talking, the circle of women went quiet. A clock ticked somewhere. Soon the meeting would be over and I wouldn't have the answers to my questions. How would I do this on my own? *Could* I do this on my own? I opened my mouth and started speaking.

'I just, um, feel like I still want to have a baby with a partner.'

There was a long pause, in which it felt like the arctic temperature dropped a few notches. Finally, a woman with an infant curled in her lap said, 'You're not ready yet.'

I wasn't ready *yet*. The sentence was revelatory. She didn't mean that I wasn't filled with enough self-love to find a soulmate. She wasn't suggesting I keep searching for love because – as per that phrase used to torture single people – *when you least expect it, you'll meet someone!* I didn't need to meditate or shed kilos or shoot Botox into the space of my third eye to win my knight. I wasn't ready, yet, to have a baby *without* a partner. The word *yet* held a promise – I was in the process of becoming ready.

After the solo mum's support meeting, Mara and I drifted over to huddle by the heater. We chatted as we wandered out to the street and decided to go for lunch. A few other women from the meeting joined us.

Over eggs in a cosy café, as Melbourne drizzled outside, I made a confession.

'I have this baby hunger,' I said. It was a phrase I'd read online. I'd written it in my journal, but never spoken it aloud.

'Me too,' the women chorused.

'Every time someone said to me, when I was trying to get pregnant, "You can have one of my kids," I wanted to punch them,' said Mara. 'It's like, I was trying so hard to have a baby, I'd done all these rounds of IVF.' She shook her head. 'They just didn't get it. They didn't know how lucky they were.' From Mara's lap, her six-month-old Rose was staring at me.

'Can I hold her?' I asked.

'Of course, please, she's getting heavy.' Mara passed Rose over to me. I took the featherweight of Rose in my arms and felt my body soften as she lay on my chest.

'I feel like people are always telling me how hard it is to have a baby on my own ... Like they disapprove,' I said.

'Anyone who tells you not to have a baby on your own can fuck off,' said Mara. We started giggling. Something started to dissolve within me.

'I mean, I don't really care what the general public thinks but my mum told me women who do this are selfish,' I explained. 'And I'm going to need my parents' support if I go through with this.'

Mara took a sip of her coffee. 'My parents were worried too. They just need time. Remember how long you were thinking about it before you made the decision. Your parents have to, like, let go of what they thought your life would be, just like you did.'

Rose's tiny fist gripped my finger as though in confirmation of what her mother had said. 'And everyone loves a baby,' Mara said. 'You'd have to have a heart of stone not to love a baby once it arrives, no matter how it was made.'

Mara took out her phone and flicked through photos. 'That's my family.' She showed us her screen. Her daughter surrounded by blue-eyed cousins and aunts and uncles and grandparents. 'Does this look like a child who needs more love?' she asked. 'This is our village, which is how it should be, that's how kids should be raised.'

'How did you make the decision?' I asked. Mara sat back in her seat and tilted her chin to the ceiling, thinking. 'I always knew,' she said slowly, 'that I wanted a baby more than I wanted a partner. A partner was never that important to me. I didn't want to have to wait.'

This echoed what I'd heard other women say in the meeting. How self-possessed these women were; how certain. Many of them younger and wiser than I, having made the decision by their early thirties. I felt envious of their conviction, the way they had shrugged off the supposed necessity of romance.

Later, as we were leaving, Mara said, 'Let's start a messaging group.' I pulled out my phone and created a group with infant emojis as its title.

As the rain started to pound down outside, Mara offered to throw my bicycle in the back of her red jeep. I gladly accepted. As she drove me home, I thought, *Maybe I won't be alone after all.*

Confession

My breath was in my throat. My heart was a canary's heart – beating at a frenzied pace. I'd decided, after the solo mum's meeting, to let my last good eggs sober up but I took a small sip of chardonnay from a fat, gleaming glass. My family and I were having lunch upstairs at a restaurant overlooking the grey sea and the smokestacks of Port Phillip Bay.

It was a perfect lunch with charred fish arranged on the plates with sauce drizzled on top but my voice was stoppered in my throat. I'd planned what I was going to say but I couldn't bring myself to say it. Should I wait for dessert so I could leave shortly afterwards and cry on my own? Or should I get it out of the way at the beginning of the meal and hope I had an appetite by dessert?

My brother Nick had flown down from Sydney with his fiancé Ellen, an elegant redhead he'd met on his first Tinder date. Nick was the only one stubborn enough to take on my mother. He was here as my armour. He was also my witness – holding me accountable to what I'd promised to say. And I had to say it, because if I was going to do this, I'd need my parents' support.

I was terrified but I heard the words coming out of my mouth, as though someone else was speaking them.

'So I've decided to have a baby on my own.'

The table was silent. We were all waiting for the person whose opinion mattered the most to us to speak. My mum. Her face had turned sour. I felt ashamed, like a small child who had broken a precious ornament.

'Are you going to have a black baby?' Mum asked.

The table exploded with laughter at the strangeness of this response, the release of a dam breaking.

We were all speaking over each other.

'What are you talking about?' Nick chided my mum.

'Are you asking her not to do that?' Ellen was puzzled.

'Didn't Sam have a black baby?' Mum said by way of explanation.

'If you have a baby of another race, and there's no father, how can they identify with their heritage?' Dad was asking.

'Sam's donor was Dominican, not that it should matter,' I said.

'No, of course not,' said Mum, 'I was just curious.'

Finally, Nick shut it down. 'I don't think this is the point. Ally is trying to tell you something.'

There was another silence. My mother's sour expression remained. She was disappointed. I was a failure. What would she say now?

'I think it could be exciting,' I offered into the void.

'I'm excited,' said Ellen, bless her.

'I'm excited,' said Nick.

'I think it's exciting,' said my dad, almost apologetically.

'And,' I said looking at my brother, 'Nick said he'd move back to Melbourne if I have a baby.'

Ellen gave Nick a flicker of a look. Maybe I shouldn't have brought that up.

'Well I'm excited about that,' said my mum.

And the conversation was closed.

I could have cried. I could have roared. I could have screamed, but I might never stop. Thankfully, the waiter appeared and cleared away the silence.

In retrospect, there were so many things I wish I'd said. I wish I'd explained myself. Told them why I'd made the decision. Framed it with the heartache and the questioning, and all the ways I had tried to find love so I could have a baby the conventional way. *I've worked so hard to get here*, I could have said. *Don't you see?* But I think I hoped they knew all that without having to say it.

'I don't want to have to brook your opposition to this,' I told my mum on the phone a few days later.

'I'm not opposing you,' she said in a voice that suggested she wasn't approving either.

'It doesn't feel like you're supporting the idea.'

'I didn't say that I don't support the idea.'

'I really need you and Dad on board, if I'm going to do this.'

'I know you do,' she said, which didn't answer the question.

On the way home from lunch in a cab, I chatted to the friendly driver. I mentioned that I was swearing off alcohol.

'Why's that?' he asked.

'I'm trying to stay healthy,' I explained. 'I want to have a baby.'

The driver instantly lit up. It was as though Hope had entered the car and sat with us, a third passenger.

When I got out, the driver turned to me, sincere: 'The next time I see you, I hope you're pregnant.'

I swallowed this kindness, grateful.

As I raked through my bag for my keys in the dim light of dusk, I thought about how this man, this driver, had given me a kind of beneficence. A belief in my future baby. A belief in me as a mother, no matter how I got there.

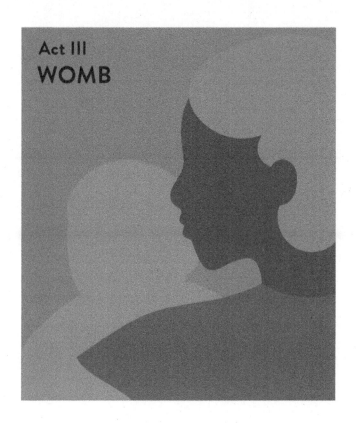

Act III
WOMB

Liberation

Once I'd made the decision to try for solo motherhood, I felt as though I had travelled to a different continent. I'd left the land of romantic fantasy where the soulmate and father of my unborn children lived. I was embarking on my own future – setting events in motion without the need for a man's approval or permission or love. It was a revelation. It was a relief. It was liberation.

It was impossible. To do this without a man, I needed some sperm.

In one hand my friend's dog yanked at the leash, and in the other I pressed the phone to my ear, as a man talked at me. The dog was dragging me past the graffitied walls along the train line, where bike riders zoomed by, getting both our hackles up. I was trying to listen intently for warning signs in the man's conversation, while dodging the real-world dangers around me.

'I've always wanted to donate sperm, but my girlfriend didn't want me to,' the man on the phone, who I'll call Sean, said. 'But now that we've broken up, I can do whatever I like.' He chuckled.

I was talking to a stranger whose life matter might end up inside me. A person whose DNA could intertwine with mine to form a speck that could grow into a creature and then become a person who would walk through the world, forever belonging to our genetic lineage.

Sean and I had connected on an app for single people or couples wanting to make a baby but lacking in sperm, eggs or a surrogate. It was designed like a dating app but, instead of a partner, I could swipe to find myself a sperm donor. Each user's profile was accompanied by cartoon icons of what the user had to offer: wiggly sperm or blobby eggs, as though we were all making babies in a children's book.

In the past, in the evenings in our share house as Lucie and I half-watched TV, I'd swiped through Tinder. Now I cautiously swiped through this app. I thumbed my way past profiles with men's photos, and others with only mountain-scapes or dawn-lit oceans. There was something worrying about this anonymity – what were these men hiding or who were they hiding from? 'What's this about?' I held the screen up to Lucie to show her an image of an empty beach where there should have been a photo of a man.

'I dunno. Maybe he's an incel?' Lucie suggested.

Ugh. I swiped onwards.

I'd written my own profile carefully – trying to present an image of myself as responsible yet creative, leaning more on my paid advertising work than my playwriting. I stated that I was surrounded by a supportive family with means – which was partly true. The full story was that since I'd told my parents my intentions, we'd avoided the subject. My profile stated that I was single yet happily independent. I was open to staying connected to the donor, but I wasn't looking to co-parent.

Writing this profile took time – it was a seduction of a different sort to online dating. I was presenting myself not as a girlfriend or wife but as a mother. A person who would be seen as mentally stable, financially and emotionally secure, firmly rooted to family and friends. I was the ideal repository for your sperm; the perfect mother of your future progeny. I was a woman who would ask nothing more from you than the time and burst of sexual energy it would take to produce and deliver your semen. Which, in truth, was all that some men required from online dating.

When I'd arrived at Sean's photo, I'd thought he looked kind. He had grey hair, a gentle smile. There was something stylish in the cut of his jacket and the filter on his profile shot. He hadn't posted many photos but his communication had been friendly and responsive. He lived interstate, which was also appealing, making it less likely that he would be involved as a parent and seek custody of a future child – which he could do, even if we signed a contract.

A landmark case involving a donor had gone to Australia's High Court. A man had donated sperm to a single woman and subsequently played an active role in his child's life. The mother had since partnered up with a woman and the couple wanted to move overseas. But the donor contested. He was named a legal parent and received court-awarded time with the child, and the woman and her partner were prevented from moving overseas. It was a thorny case that had no doubt been painful for all sides. The case had echoes of the long history of discrimination against lesbian couples and the prevailing belief that a child needed a father. But there was a legal precedent, nonetheless, and it was a path I wanted to avoid.

'I'm coming down to Melbourne soon, sometime in the next few weeks,' Sean said. The dog and I arrived at the park, it was yanking at my arm socket to be released into the grassy carpet of smells. I unclipped the leash and it was away.

'I'll take you out to dinner when I come to town,' Sean said.

I felt a sharp twinge in my neck. This sounded suspiciously like a date.

∾

Now that I was looking for donor sperm, it seemed improbable that women fell pregnant by accident. 'Just go down to the pub and have a one-night stand,' people said to me – and to every person with a womb I knew, lesbians included, who had considered solo motherhood. It was a cheaper option than buying donor sperm from a clinic. But the solo mothers I knew had forged this path with studious intentionality. A pub shag was the opposite of intentional. It didn't take into account the health and safety risks of sex with a stranger, or if (and it was a big *if*) you got pregnant, what you would tell your future child. Would you even remember her father's name? Or you might be bound to co-parent with a stranger for the rest of your life – a guy who might have looked appealing after three beers in the semi-dark of the sticky-carpeted pub on a Friday night but would be dangerously less so when entrusted with caring for the soft, imprintable life of a baby.

No. Absolutely not. A pub shag was out of the question. It

was impossible for me to reverse back along the tightrope I had walked to get to this point.

I envied that imaginary woman who could go to a bar – blind to consequence and her own intentions. She could look across the room and see another person – a flicker of recognition passing between them; an acknowledgement that she and this unknown man would gradually move their bodies closer over the course of the night. After several drinks, leaning against a damp wall in a cobbled laneway, they would close the space between their mouths, pouring themselves into one another. Later still, in an unfamiliar room, she would step clean out of her clothes and exchange flakes of skin and sweat and hot breath and the slosh of bodily fluid with a stranger. Then two weeks later find herself (*Oh shit! How did this happen?*) … pregnant.

A stranger was too risky. A data bank of men from a fertility clinic – which weren't accompanied by photos – seemed too anonymous. I liked the idea of having sperm donated by someone I knew. Sperm from a friend or someone I could get to know on an app seemed preferable to a donor code on an administrative file. I wanted a man whose face I could study, whose kindness I could measure in its creases. Also, at the time one vial of donor sperm was upwards of $2000 – that was before medications and procedures and the potential for multiple rounds of treatment and maybe even IVF in future (around $10,000 per cycle) were factored in. I had recently found myself a regular writing gig which would pay for the treatment but I didn't have any savings if it didn't work the first time. I was adamant that I would not ask my parents for money and I doubted they would have lent it to me to pursue this path.

There were casual offers from men I knew. One night a married friend had said, 'I'll help you out. You can have my sperm, if you want it.' He exhaled on his joint, while his wife looked on, unsure how to react. I smiled and thanked him. But I knew I wouldn't take him up on it. His face was prematurely weathered by his love of the good life – wine, pot, drugs – and while I adored him, I suspected his predilections may be addictions.

I confided in my friend Serge about my predicament. Each week, Serge and I met to dance in the dark in a large church hall in Melbourne's inner north surrounded by a hundred other bodies. Afterwards, we walked through the chilly evening, sweat cooling on our backs.

I had never forgotten the words he had said to me years earlier after we had kissed one drunken evening. 'I don't want a baby and you'll never convince me to have one with you.' The reasons veered between him being too old (he was nearing forty-five) and the climate crisis.

Now he had a girlfriend who had children, and things had shifted between Serge and me to a safer zone. We had travelled through that romantic obstacle to the other side. It was all behind us.

'So, I'm planning to try to have a baby using donor sperm,' I said as we made our way down the silent, terraced streets.

'Wow, OK.' He took it in, nodding. 'Whose sperm are you going to use?'

'I haven't figured that out yet.'

'Well, my genes are excellent. My family have a great lineage,' he laughed. 'You can have my sperm if you want.'

My mouth opened and closed in shock.

'But you told me that you never want to have children!' I was confused.

'This is different. And don't you want a donor who can babysit occasionally?'

I didn't know what to say. I was elated. This could be the ideal solution.

I took Serge's offer away to think about it. Serge was healthy and fit; he had a sharp intellect and a fierce curiosity. I loved the meeting of our minds, the way he generously laughed at my jokes and was always on board for whatever adventure I suggested. He could be the perfect donor. Maybe a happy friendship was exactly what you needed for a melding of genes.

A week later, Serge and I met again to dance in the dark. We separated off into different spaces – he at the back of the hall behind all the bodies ('White men can't dance,' he would joke) and me on the parquetry near the front. I loved the freedom I felt when moving wildly to the music, with no concern for coordination, as the outlined bodies floated by in the dark hall.

Afterwards, we walked to a nearby bar and ordered hot toddies. A nervous current of electricity infinitely looped from my chest to my guts. We sat on stools at a high table, sipping our drinks.

'How's your hot toddy?' I asked, wondering when it was best to bring up his offer of sperm.

'Mmm. It needs more lemon,' Serge said, screwing his face up. 'And more honey. And more whisky.' We laughed.

I was holding the mug close, the warmth spreading through my chest and hands. Up until that minute, my drink had seemed perfectly fine. Now I looked down and instead of a hot toddy, I saw a baby wedged against my heart. I could sense Serge frowning at the baby, and the way I was inexpertly holding it. I'd forgotten how critical Serge could be.

'So about the sperm thing,' Serge said.

I looked up at him. The baby was gone.

'I talked to my girlfriend about it, and I'm sorry, but I don't think I can do it. She's not comfortable with it. If I was single ...' he raised his hands in apology.

I took a sip of my drink.

I understood. If my boyfriend had offered to donate sperm to a close single friend, I'd feel wary. Serge was still talking and everything he was saying made sense – how complicated it would be, how it opened up questions about the nature of our relationship.

'And she wanted to know how I'd deliver the sperm.' Serge grinned, raising his eyebrows, and letting out a brief laugh – the implication of sex hanging in the air.

'Huh,' I said. *I'm not planning to fuck you*, I didn't say.

I was disappointed and relieved. It was never going to be as simple as Serge handing over his sperm. We had a complicated history. I felt stupid for thinking it would be straightforward.

If I'd become pregnant with Serge's sperm, I would have to weather his exacting standards and all the ways he drove me crazy. And we weren't in love, so why would I do that? Why would I wed myself to another person, someone I felt a deep affection for but who wasn't my partner? How could I do something as life altering as having a baby with him?

But now there was Sean on the app – who might be someone with less strings. On the phone, Sean had laid out his assets –

he had a daughter, a good job, the ability to jump on a plane interstate whenever he liked and pick up the tab for dinner. 'I'll take you somewhere nice,' he said with cavalier largesse. His sperm, it seemed, was just another gift – a baby, like a generous tip, added to the tab.

I wandered around the damp, well-trodden patch of the dog park, smiling at the familiar faces of the other dog owners after I'd hung up from the call with Sean. I took out my phone and googled his name. I pulled up a LinkedIn profile. Found a photo of his daughter. Everything he said checked out. But there was something else.

The way Sean talked was familiar. A cloud drifted away to reveal the blanched sun and a beam of clarity.

Sean didn't want to be a donor. He was looking for a woman who could give him a baby, add to his assets – a woman who could expand his family portfolio. Sean wanted a wife. I found it strange, slightly creepy even, that Sean thought a baby-making app was the place to find his match. Or perhaps he was doing this seduction act to multiple women, more women than he should. Each state had family limits that donors at clinics were supposed to abide by. There was no way to police this outside of the clinics but the spirit of the law was clear in its intention: to protect future children from being related to hundreds of siblings. How many women was Sean donating sperm to?

Meeting up with Sean might also be dangerous. While my profile clearly stated artificial insemination as my method of sperm delivery, there were warnings on the VARTA website about women reporting being pressured or harassed into sex or sexually assaulted by informal donors.

I needed to go back to the idea of a friend – someone I trusted. Maybe even someone who I could live a modern, utopian, co-parenting ideal with. And why just one man, when I could have two?

I had long fantasised that my friends Seb and Evan – a gay couple – would be excellent co-parents if I ever planned to have a baby alone. They now had a surrogate child of their own – from overseas – a baby who had been many years and thousands of dollars and kilometres of travel in the making. I envied their life of stability and warmth and I loved them dearly as friends. Perhaps now that they had one child, they would want a sibling for their daughter? One that was shared with an old friend, rather than finding a surrogate.

I imagined an idyllic scenario where I lived in the house next door to Seb and Evan and we all raised our baby. A home where multiple parents and grandparents tripped in and out providing for our baby with the hands of many, instead of just one. That we could share the ardour and the arduous tasks of parenthood. I knew it would be a marriage of sorts but why not? They were kind and steady, excellent fathers and dear friends, and there would be no romantic confusion between us.

We would have a modern-day *Tales of the City*, that iconic series of books set in San Francisco's late 1970s, with an eclectic community living around a communal courtyard on Barbary Lane. In my version there would be less partying and more baby laundry. It was a dream: more love for my baby, more help, more family. A life filled with an abundance of people and comfort and togetherness. My own family had always been small and distant, with only a handful of cousins. I was greedy for more of what I'd never had.

After months of deliberation, I got on a train and headed north to visit Seb and Evan. To anyone who glanced over, I looked like an ordinary person sitting on a train – not a woman who was holding her heart in her hands. Through the window, as I moved closer to my destination, I watched the sky widen over the low buildings, and the trees became sparse streaks between the roads. I'd been rehearsing in my mind what I would say.

'I feel like I need to make a compelling pitch,' I'd explained to Lucie over breakfast at a café a few days before. She screwed up her face at the word *pitch* with its salesy connotations, as though I was a sperm Svengali.

'I feel like I need to sell them on it,' I said.

'I don't think you want to *sell* them,' Lucie sounded disapproving. I felt flustered and annoyed. She didn't understand.

'I just need to plan it, you know?' I could see that the more words I spoke the further I was travelling from her. This was what I was afraid would happen with Seb and Evan. That words would fail me.

In Seb and Evan's chic, minimalist living room, I played with my friends' happy, apple-cheeked baby. She crawled towards me over the sunlight-dappled carpet as I shook a rattle to lure her. She grabbed the rattle and her mouth opened into a gummy smile. I wanted to eat her whole.

Seb and Evan and I chatted about this and that and nothing in particular. How good a sleeper their daughter, Emma, was, and eater too. There was a familiar whirring up my spine: my old friend anxiety. *Say it. Say it now.* I was about to make a proposal. To get my soul on bended knee and ask for the impossible, to reveal my most tender, naked want.

I feigned casual. 'So I'm, um, planning on having a baby on my own with a sperm donor.'

'That's incredible,' said Seb.

'So fantastic, good on you,' said Evan. 'We highly recommend the whole parenting thing.'

Their beams buoyed me on.

'Thanks. And I, ah, wondered if you'd want a sibling for Emma?'

I didn't say: Will you be my sperm donor? I didn't say: Could we raise a child together? I didn't say: I want this more than anything in the world.

I didn't need to. My friends intuited my meaning. There was a pause where I felt my chest cave in. Thankfully neither Seb nor Evan looked at each other. 'I think,' Seb said carefully, 'we'd want to do it as a family.'

'Of course,' I said, trying to lift the corners of my mouth into a smile.

I left soon after, hurrying down their front path, past their garden brimming with fat green natives that had been lovingly grown. *Stupid idiot.* Even though I hadn't spoken the words, I'd humiliated myself. As the metal gate swung shut behind me, so did their family.

Donor

On the phone, I could hear the exhaustion in Mara's voice after having wrestled Rose, her eight-month-old, to sleep for the last hour on her own. We spoke and texted now all the time. Mara was walking ahead on the same path, and her wisdom illuminated the shadowy parts of this life I was making.

I was telling Mara about my adventures on the baby app and my failed attempt to find the right friend to donate sperm.

'Have you looked at using a clinic donor?' Mara asked.

I sighed. 'Yeah, but don't you think it's weird that when you go with a clinic-recruited donor there's no photo? Like what if they're ugly or … ' I didn't finish the sentence; I didn't need to.

'Hang on,' said Mara. I waited as Mara listened for her baby's cries then there was a staticky scrape as she pushed her phone back to her ear. 'Sorry, false alarm. Yeah, I know what you mean about the clinic not having photos, I remember feeling worried about that. But once I had Rose, it didn't matter who the donor was. You just love your baby. I never think: *Oh, I wish I'd used a different donor.* Being her mum kinda feels like it was meant to be.'

Meant to be. A baby. How badly I wanted those things.

'I just thought I'd know the donor – that maybe I'd see his face, get to know him … that we'd be friends,' I said.

'Yeah, but it's the same problem as finding a guy. You've already made the decision to go solo so why complicate that? A clinic donor means that you get to choose. You make the decisions. You're in control. And it's just waaaay safer.'

After we hung up, I scrolled through article after article online featuring pixelated blurred men and women and I realised how naïve I'd been about the unregulated world of donor conception. There were stories of children who had found out that they were one of a litter, with hundreds of other siblings. There were unregulated male donors who claimed to be psychologically and medically sound but were not. There were men who wanted to scatter their seed across the world and populate it with their children in a sick, macho show of prowess. There were donor-conceived adults who didn't realise, until too late, that they had married their sibling. Soul-wrenching tales of people whose selfhood had been blown to bits by the truth of their making and their biology.

On Facebook, there were groups like the confusingly named Australia Backpackers Seeking Sperm Donation. Their About section read: 'We get many backpacker men wishing to donate and have a couple of children while travelling Australia. You can arrange petrol and travel money from your recipients and accommodation while they're trying to conceive.' I pictured these men wandering along dusty highways – with their sperm and a swag – exchanging a future human for a feed and a night of shelter.

It was clear that some donors and doctors – usually with the best of intentions – despite their goal to make humans, hadn't considered the very-human consequences. The consequences were small, beating fleshy hearts walking around the world, the consequence was a real child who deserved to grow up knowing who they were, to be able to know their donor and their siblings. They deserved to have an intact identity, not one diluted by being one of hundreds of offspring; to know they weren't made in exchange for a night of accommodation or some cash. Parents and donor-conceived children deserved to have all the information possible from the start about their safe, screened and healthy donors.

The medical profession had played a very dubious part in the history of donor conception. But the men who donated to fertility clinics in Australia now had to undergo a series of screening tests (such as HIV tests, genetic testing and sperm count) and two counselling sessions. Their sperm was tested, then quarantined and retested three months later to properly check for transmissible diseases. The process was more thorough and safe than unregulated donor conception. There were legal contracts in place to protect everyone involved, which prevented the donor from making parentage claims or the recipient making child support claims. The clinic donors had to abide by the family limits (no more than ten families total, including the donor's own, in Victoria and most Australian states, and five families total in others). This ensured the child wouldn't end up being related to hundreds of others. In my state, clinic donors were also recorded on a formal register run by VARTA (and in other states, fertility clinics were legally required to keep those records).

While it would cost money to go through a clinic, I would be paying for a larger degree of freedom, safety and security. In future, my child would have access to VARTA's counselling service in the process of connecting with their donor. There would be structures in place to protect and support them.

There were so many ways to fuck up as a parent after your kid was born. But in the process of choosing a donor, I could try my best to protect my child. The internet was a murky and risky place to find sperm. I shut down Facebook and called Melbourne IVF to pay for access to the donor database.

I logged on to the Melbourne IVF database and sifted through the small pool of donors. I had roughly ten men to choose from. The donors were categorised by procedure – IVF sperm, which is united with an egg in a petri dish outside the woman's body, is different from sperm used for insemination, which requires speedy swimmers. As a woman who just scraped under forty, with no known fertility issues, I would first have to pay for the full cost of two rounds of IUI (intrauterine insemination) before I could qualify for Medicare rebated IVF.

The donors at the clinic were provided without their names or identifying details (such as date of birth). But they weren't strictly anonymous like they had been in the past; they were 'identity release' donors. This meant that although the name and identifying details were not stated on a donor's profile, once a child was born, the parent or donor-conceived child could apply for that information from the Victorian central register at the age of eighteen (or younger, if a counsellor gave approval).

I logged in and out of the donor database over a series of weeks, with a prickling sensation in my fingertips, my breath shallow. I read and re-read the letters the men had to provide to their potential offspring. There were no photos – my search predated some clinics introducing baby pictures of the donors. All I had to go on were the characteristics that the donor had written in a neat hand, like eye and hair colour and physical build.

How could I make such a monumental choice based on such scant information? These men were stick figure outlines. A few pages could never adequately convey their depth and complexity. How would I know which one was the right choice to be the biological father of my child? And none of the men stood out to me – I dismissed them for petty things: grammar mistakes or bad taste in music. They all left me feeling lukewarm and indecisive.

It was strange to know so little about this man who could be providing half the genetic material for my child – to not even be able to see a picture of his face. But I kept replaying Mara's words: *You just love your baby.* Despite my doubts, it still seemed like magic. I could choose one of these donors and have *my baby*.

Sifting through the donor profiles, I opened up a profile I hadn't read. As I speed-read, I felt my face get hot: he was a film director, he was artistic, he was open-minded. I could barely breathe. He was exactly the kind of intelligent, creative guy that I would be attracted to. This was a match, I knew it. I was in love.

I flicked through his profile again and let out a groan when I saw it: he was an IVF donor, not an IUI donor, which meant I couldn't use his sperm, at least not until my two rounds of insemination had failed. This was not my man. I logged out, dejected, and moped through the next week feeling as though I'd been dumped.

In my journal, I wrote lists of things to do. Of practicalities that I needed to take care of in order to have a child.

Choose a donor.

Do a budget.

Find somewhere to live on my own.

I was still living in a share house with Lucie and another housemate. It was hardly the ideal place to raise a baby. Lucie was planning to buy a place soon on her own with her hard-earned teacher's savings and my other housemate was moving in with her boyfriend. And I planned to move across the city, to be closer to my parents because hopefully, ideally, they would be able to help me out with the baby. While my brother Nick had offered to move to Melbourne if I had a baby, he had a life in Sydney. He was getting married and hoping to start a family of his own. I couldn't rely on him being around. I still thought of my youngest brother, Tom, as the baby, even though he was in his late twenties, and I wasn't sure I could count on him for help. This brought me to the last item on my list:

Talk to Mum and Dad about childcare (argh!).

Choosing a donor seemed easier than talking to my parents about what kind of grandparenting help they could give me in the future. But it needed to be done.

A few weeks later, we were celebrating dinner for my dad's birthday in a new restaurant across from the botanical gardens. My brother Tom and I sat across from my parents.

A cute Irish waiter in a slate-coloured pinafore apron with matching eyes was flirting with the table. *Focus*, I told myself. This was no time to get distracted. The waiter left. I laid out my dilemma to my parents.

'So I wanted to talk to you, at some point, not right now, about childcare. When I have a baby, I'd really love your help.

Because I'll be the sole earner, I'm going to need to work so …
If you could think about whether you'd be open to doing any
regular babysitting. We don't have to talk about it now but if
you could have a think.' I stopped talking, gulped some water.
Waited.

'We can talk about it *if* you have a baby,' Mum said, as though
that definitely wasn't going to happen. I felt the furious whine of a
teenage girl bubbling up inside me. *Breathe*, I told myself.

'I need to plan, Mum. I'm trying to be sensible about this. To
do a budget and figure out childcare in advance.'

'Four hours a week,' Mum said in a clipped staccato.

Tom and I glanced at each other bemused.

'You can think about it,' I attempted.

'A day a week,' my mum said, as though she was bargaining
with an invisible opponent, but in reverse.

My brother shook his head.

'We're getting old,' Dad said, 'so we can't do too much.'

'We're almost seventy,' Mum agreed.

'Most grandparents we know only do a day a week,' Dad said
as though I was disagreeing with him.

I wasn't sure why this felt like an argument. Perhaps, for my
parents, agreeing to help with childcare felt like a slippery slope
towards condoning my choice. It didn't feel like they were saying
no to childcare, but their response held no guarantee either.

The table quietened as the flirty waiter poured us more wine.
When he left, my mother asked in a lowered voice.

'When are you planning to do fertility treatment?'

'Well, I was going to start next month, but I've got that trip
and I don't think it's going to be easy to carry the drugs on a

plane. The doctor said they need to be refrigerated. So I'm going to wait another month.'

'Oh good,' Mum said. 'That gives you a month to meet your knight in shining armour.'

I looked from my fiercely intelligent, capable mother to my father.

'So Dad's your knight in shining armour, is he?' I scoffed.

'Of course, he is,' she said, as though I was mad to suggest otherwise.

When I got home from dinner, I opened up the donor database and sifted through the men's profiles to see if there was anyone new. Who were these men, I wondered, who decided to donate their sperm? What drove them to do it? Was it ego, kindness, desire, longing?

I clicked on each man's profile again and re-read them to see if there was anything I'd missed. If there'd been a shopping cart, I would have dragged men in there and left them for days on end. 'You haven't completed your sperm purchase!' the marketing emails would read. I snapped my laptop shut, still undecided.

The next morning I logged back in to find a shiny 'New Donor' flag next to one of the options. I read his profile, noted that he wasn't a genetic carrier for cystic fibrosis as I am, that he seemed kind enough, healthy enough, athletic and thoughtful enough. What was I waiting for?

This was a man who I'd never have to watch eat breakfast noisily, his mouth agape. This was a man who wouldn't fall asleep during a date. This was a man who wouldn't lecture me about how a keto diet really can cure depression.

My finger hovered over the 'proceed with this donor' button. I took a long inhale, held my breath and clicked my mouse. It was done: the website immediately barred access after choosing a donor. I had a two-month deadline to begin treatment as there were a limited number of donors in the pool for women to use. Two months for my eggs to meet their match.

How strange. How wondrous. How clinical. I was floating. If this worked, I'd just chosen the biological father of my child.

Treatment

'We're just going to get this done,' my new fertility specialist Kate Stern said as I sat in her office to go through the treatment plan. Kate had a way of moving while sitting still, her whole body buzzed, her strawberry curls bouncing, her eyes electric as they sparked green and hazel. 'Head down, bum up!' she declared as though she was a footy coach giving a rallying speech. Despite Kate's optimism, my chances of getting pregnant through insemination at the age of thirty-nine were around 15 to 18 per cent.

After the appointment, a nurse talked me through the follicle stimulating hormone injections. 'You'll do one injection each morning,' she said breezily. I anxiously watched as she showed me how to fit the needle to the vial. Next to me sat a small cooler bag I'd been instructed to bring with me for the medication. These expensive elixirs required refrigeration.

I felt like Jack with his magic beans as I picked up the bag carefully. The small vials with their tremoring liquid were going to travel to the shared kitchen at my writer's studio and sit silently during my day's work, until I could take them home.

Anyone could pass by the kitchen at my studio – the building was open to the public. 'I'm just worried a stranger might steal the bag,' I said to the nurse, as though the medication was like an empty car with keys in the ignition for would-be fertility bandits.

'Of course,' the nurse said, ever attentive to the wild imaginings of women undergoing fertility treatment. I watched as she placed numerous skull and crossbones *Danger* stickers on the bag to deter thieves.

I took the bag out to the street and packed it into the basket on the back of my bike. As I coasted away from the city's enclave of doctors' and dentists' offices, I hoped that the contents didn't spill out onto the road.

After a day of writing, I would ride home where I planned to hide the bag at the back of my share house fridge. Lucie knew about what I was up to, but my other housemate didn't. I wasn't ready to share my plan with the wider world yet. It felt too delicate, too unreal to speak out loud. I felt it might jinx my chances of getting pregnant.

That night, I watched the movie *Private Life*, where Kathryn Hahn and Paul Giamatti played a couple who go through fertility treatment. Hahn's belly was covered in coin-sized bruises from the hormone injections. It occurred to me after watching the film that I had no idea what I was embarking on. That I wasn't even entirely sure how my body worked – the anatomy of conception was vaguely clear, the process of follicle stimulating hormones was muddy.

It's an exciting time, Mara had texted me.

I don't feel excited. I guess because nothing's happened yet. Feels like I'm waiting to board a train, I wrote back.

I watched as the little dots on-screen danced.

It's more of a rollercoaster than a train, she replied.

In the lead-up to Christmas, I went to the acupuncturist, I jogged, I trained at the gym. I meditated. I felt like my body had become a thing to be tuned and trained and constantly improved upon. I went to a wildcrafter – a kind of naturopath-cum-witch. 'To be a mother, you need to learn how to mother yourself,' the wildcrafter told me in her gentle Canadian accent. I wondered how to do that exactly. 'Your womb is a garden,' she explained. 'You've left it quite late to tend the garden but we'll do our best.'

The wildcrafter mixed me up a sludgy brew of herbs for my womb garden that tasted like a dredged pond. As I drove home, I tried to visualise my womb, but I could only picture a rubbish heap full of weeds.

At night, before bed, I wrote letters in my journal to my yet-to-be-conceived child. *You will not be deterred by all this talk,* I wrote. *You will stick and grow. You will be mine and I will be yours. I can't wait.* Then a few days later: *There is no knowing if it will work and if it does, what terror and joy may follow.*

I was not all saintly though. The ad agency I worked for had a Christmas party which I mentally christened 'My Last Hurrah'. Even though I'd stopped drinking these last few months, if there was an event that required alcohol to be bearable it was the work Christmas party.

In the backroom of a city restaurant, with hard echoey surfaces, the chatter of my colleagues rose to a roar, induced by too much wine and too little food. I sat at a long table, feeling blanketed by tipsiness, by the safety of my smart, female colleagues around me. I turned to find my boss, Trev, taking a seat next to me. Trev was a loud, brash man in his fifties who liked to shadowbox his way through the office. 'So, Ally,' he interrupted the chatter with his booming voice. 'Do you have a partner?'

The table fell quiet. Everyone was waiting. A hot clod of embarrassment was spreading out from my chest. I considered making a joke but the silence had stretched on for too long and I was all out of jokes. 'No, I don't.' I shook my head. Trev stared at me, waiting for an explanation. Everything in me wanted to make excuses, to justify my disreputable single status. I clamped my mouth shut. *You don't have to fucking explain yourself to anyone.*

I rarely spoke about my dating life at work. And I'd been keeping my upcoming fertility treatment a secret. All of it felt like a green shoot of hope curled up inside me that had to be protected from the threshing machine of productivity and timesheets and branding jargon. Trying to conceive alone felt salacious, controversial. I wanted to keep it from my colleagues, many of whom were married with children.

After lunch, we piled into minibuses and went to a pub that had once been a dank dive but had a newly renovated polish and served espresso martinis, which I drank two of in quick succession. The air was filled with that anarchic end of year rush where colleagues who were half strangers began to show their shadow selves.

In the gleaming, black-tiled bathroom, a young graphic designer offered me a line of coke to snort off her phone, using a rupee note. I didn't like coke, or espresso martinis but it was My Last Hurrah so I went into the shiny toilet stall and snorted a line, feeling the cold chemical sting at the back of my throat.

When I emerged from the stall, the designer was bright-eyed, flying. She leant against the sinks and told me about her divorce at the age of twenty-five. 'I didn't really talk about it at work, but people knew.' Her pupils were a pinprick of brightness. I thought about what I wasn't talking about at work, the secrets I was hiding, and nodded.

A few hours later, I found myself out on the footpath just as it started pounding steamy, summer rain. Next to me were a group of kids – they must've been barely in their twenties – who shrieked drunkenly. The girls were in shrink-wrapped skirts and daggered heels, the boys in muscle t-shirts, swaying and cheering. I was suddenly old.

Two days later, after the hangover had subsided, I was restless and anxious to begin. I stared down at my belly in bed. It was flat, lifeless. I was ready to take my future into my own hands. To get on the train, or the rollercoaster, and depart. I thought of Mara. Before having her daughter, she'd been through numerous rounds of failed IVF, a missed miscarriage and a botched surgery.

Scrolling down the feed of my solo mum Facebook group, there were endless threads detailing disappointing IVF cycles. A dark inventory trailed many of these women: ectopic pregnancies, endometriosis, the loss of fallopian tubes, IVF pregnancies with no heartbeat.

Mara had told me that she'd thought about having a second child but while she could countenance disappointment, she couldn't take on the cost – she estimated that she'd spent $43,000 on her first. And although there was a perception that women pursuing IVF were forty-something careerists with means, the solo mums I'd met in Australia spanned age and backgrounds and professions.

These women online, whose names and faces I felt affection and familiarity with, had saved money, forfeited expensive trips and nights out with friends. They had babysat other people's children on weekends to pay for treatment. They had repeatedly lived through the wait of hope and heartbreak that was stretched between embryo transfer and blood test. Their selfless actions spoke of devotion – the quality we ask of mothers.

Flicking through their stories, I wondered if I had three or six years of failed treatments in me – if I could countenance the maddening despair and the financial cost? If I would have to measure how much it was worth – to my sanity, to my bank account – to have a baby alone?

I couldn't afford more than a few rounds of IUI treatment. I'd wilfully and blindly avoided thinking too far ahead about what it could cost – about what credit could be maxed, about what lengths I would travel and debts I would shoulder to become a mother. About how the process could crush my spirit. I didn't let my mind drift to the other women I knew, the ones for whom IVF, despite years of trying and paying, had not worked. The women who were childless, and not by choice.

On 25 December 2018, the day of the Virgin birth, a dull ache in my uterus heralded the arrival of my period. Not just any period. The most highly anticipated period of my life. Soon my uterus would start to shed. Hallelujah. Praise the moon. The arrival of my period meant that I could soon begin the first cycle. I called the fertility clinic. They instructed me to start the self-administered injections in two days.

The needles, the self-stab to the gut, filled me with dread. I was cat-sitting at a friend's house a few blocks from the sea. I asked Lucie to come over to swim laps on the morning of my first injection but also for moral support. We kicked out through the emerald dark of the sea, freestyling side-by-side to the heritage pier and back. We walked home, towels around our waists, hair damp on our backs, not speaking much, my mind fogged with what was to come.

In the kitchen, I lined up the needle and the vial of drugs on the table. It was early but the summer heat was already pressing in against the windows. Lucie watched silently as I attached a needle to the pen filled with the vial of medicine. 'Hey, look at me,' Lucie said and held up her phone. I raised the needle in the air like a dagger and gave a manic, silly grin as she shot a photo. We giggled.

I pulled up my dress and pinched the skin on my belly between forefinger and thumb and tried to position the needle at the correct angle as my heart yammered. I felt the twin adrenalin surge of fear and excitement. I looked up at Lucie and then back at my abdomen. I was really doing this. I inhaled, held my breath and plunged the needle in. Stab. Two. Three. Four. I counted as I pushed down on the pen to release the hormones into my body. I felt ... nothing.

'Do you think it worked?' I asked, panicked. Lucie and I scrutinised the pen to see if the clear liquid had emptied. It was impossible to tell. I'd been prepared for pain. Now I was worried because there'd been none. I called the nurse at the clinic and explained the absence of sensation. 'Sounds about right,' she said dryly.

Each morning, I injected the low dose of the drugs into the flab beneath my belly button with the medicine-filled pen. The medication would help the one dominant follicle to grow, filled with a ripe, juicy egg ready to meet the sperm on insemination day.

On day three, I woke to a piercing pain in my lower abdomen. The word *mittelschmerz* floated into my head. 'Ovulation pain,' my mum had once explained to me as a teenager when I had mysterious, crippling pain two weeks before my period.

Oh God, was I ovulating? It was too early. I remembered Mara had missed her window by ovulating in the waiting room of the clinic and her whole cycle had been ruined. If I ovulated now it could be too late to be inseminated. All of this would be a waste. I dialled the clinic, pacing up and down in the kitchen. I explained breathlessly to the nurse what was happening. She listened calmly. 'Just keep an eye on how you're feeling and give us a call back later if the pain is still an issue.'

I went to my studio in the old convent. My room – one of the former nun's cells – was west facing, it looked out on the spires of the convent built at the turn of the nineteenth century, and to a courtyard with an ancient liquidambar tree. The heat in the afternoons was unbearable, so I pulled the blind halfway down and worked in the semi-dark. I had scenes to write for my musical that had to be finished. In five months' time, I was planning to fly to New York for rehearsals and the Off Broadway production. I wasn't sure how a possible pregnancy would fit in with this plan but I had to continue living towards other ambitions, to hold parallel futures in my mind. Pregnant or not pregnant. The writing gave me a way to be somewhere else – a conduit to another world. And working when everyone else was holidaying between Christmas and New Year made me feel pure and untouchable. After a few hours, I noticed that the pain in my abdomen had mysteriously ebbed away.

I rode my bike home, bumping through a cobbled laneway littered with sodden cardboard and debris, when a man rode up beside me. 'Hello,' he said. I felt the air sharpen, his shadow heavy and close. Then I realised that it was Buddy, Lucie's cousin.

'You scared the shit out of me, Buddy,' I yelled.

'Oh God, I'm so sorry.' He laughed and then I did too and we were both gasping for air, laughing hysterically.

Buddy was almost a decade younger than Lucie. He was tall and lean with shaved hair to hide his baldness and swirls of elegant tattoos along his arms. He spoke nervously, the way he always had, ever since I'd known him as a teenager, his eyes skittering away from mine.

We rode home together and he told me about his recent year overseas, how he'd dated then broken up with his girlfriend who was either French or Dutch, I couldn't remember. I'd glimpsed her online once: stunning and willowy and impossibly chic.

We got to the turnoff to his place but Buddy offered to ride me to my door. When we got there, he sat on his bike, propping it against my fence.

'Sorry I've just blabbed nonstop, what's happening with you?' he asked.

'Um, well nothing, or everything, I guess. I'm trying to get pregnant. Using a sperm donor.' I felt shy saying the words.

'What? That's rad. I wish I could do that,' he said.

'What do you mean, have a baby or get pregnant?' I asked.

'I dunno, just being able to grow a baby seems …' He shook his head. 'I'd just like to have a kid one day and I imagine that being able to create one from your own body … I wish I could experience that.'

This was not the reaction I'd had from other male friends. There was something about Buddy, I thought, as he waved at me and rode away under the sun, which was dipping its way beneath the concrete warehouses.

The next day, I drove down to the coast to see Sam's family and her barely four-month-old donor-conceived success story: her son Loki. When I arrived, Sam's mum, a bright-eyed brunette, folded me into her arms in a warm hug. Sam's family was large and loud – the four sisters cackled and shrieked together as we played board games along with her parents each night. They were a stark contrast to my family. When my family went away together in the summer, each of us were often wrapped up in our thoughtful, anxious silences, quietly reading books in hammocks or separate nooks of the house.

Two summers before, walking along the beach as the waves tumbled and churned ceaselessly, Sam had told her mum that she wanted to become a solo parent. Her mum had started to cry. 'I don't want you to give up,' she'd said. Then within minutes, her mum had changed course, pragmatic: 'I'll have to retire so I can help raise the baby.' Sam's close-knit family, her sisters and parents, had supported her decision from the start. I longed for a family like Sam's. While my brothers were on board and knew that I'd started treatment, I hadn't yet told my parents.

As we sat in the backyard, the bundle of baby Loki was passed around each day from family member to family member and then on to me. He sat in my lap, staring up at me with a worried frown. It was time for him to feed. I passed him to Sam. She was struggling to produce breastmilk. Her face was pale and splotched from lack of sleep. 'We're getting there,' she winced as Loki tried to latch, eyeing the world around him suspiciously. Sam was handed a pint of Guinness – that promised elixir for stimulating breastmilk. 'Now, we're getting there.' Sam grinned and raised her glass.

I was watching Sam's new life carefully to see how my own might unfold. She was cheerful but I could sense a struggle beneath the surface – her former life of independence now eclipsed by the bewilderment and exhaustion of solo motherhood.

On day five, I took the cooler bag out of the fridge. No one in Sam's family paid any attention to my injections. 'Don't worry, no one is going to touch your drugs,' Sam's mum joked as she swung the fridge open, 'we're only after the cheese.'

On New Year's Eve, we sat outside and I had a glass of champagne. A pregnant friend and her husband sat at the end of the table. She was a few months away from giving birth, her swollen belly like an attachment to her slim body. Later, we watched through a fence as a few fireworks fizzled above an open field. Below, clumps of families stood with their faces tilted towards the night sky. I closed my eyes for a second and tried to hold the sparking light behind my eyelids, praying a godless prayer for it to bring me a new life in the new year.

On the seventh day of treatment, back in Melbourne, I went to the clinic for a scan. Kate pointed at one of my follicles – a small black circle surrounded by white flecks of cloud. 'Eighteen millimetres,' she said. 'And your lining looks good. I'm going to give you a trigger injection for tonight.'

I was stunned. Tonight? I had tickets booked to a show for Lucie's birthday. Kate shrugged. The trigger, she explained, would make my hormones surge so that I ovulated in roughly 40 hours. They would inseminate me on Friday, before the weekend. *Oh God, this is happening, it's really happening.*

I knew that if this worked, if I got pregnant, I would feel like everything up to this moment was ordained. As I left my appointment, the trigger injection loaded in my cooler bag, my mind unfurled back through the years of dating, of agonised decision-making, through hundreds of sunrises in reverse, then flew backwards through the sky to New York and that morning in bed with Dave, where everything ended and began.

That night, I sat in the dark theatre next to Lucie, unable to focus on the musical I was watching. Onstage the actors were dashing around in slapstick fashion and radiating exuberance. The audience were laughing and whooping but I felt like I was underwater. I kept checking the time on my phone, surreptitiously pressing the button in my lap.

At 9.10 pm, I snuck out, a dark shadow sliding along the aisle, clutching a small bright-yellow cooler bag. Through the bathroom door, I heard the muffled honky tonk of the piano onstage and the chorus resounding through the packed theatre.

I had planned to go into a stall but it was too cramped to comfortably inject myself. I propped my phone on the sink and waited for the exact minute to tick over. The timing was important – the injection was not to be too early or too late so that the egg perished or the sperm missed its window and fizzled to nothing. As I stood poised, needle above my naked waist, I felt a thrill of purpose run through me, a wonder at being able to steer my body's fate.

If anyone had walked into the bathroom, they would have seen a woman, jumpsuit stripped down to her waist, in her bra with a large white pen, like a teacher's marker, with a needle on its tip. The phone glowed: 9.20 pm. I pushed down on the trigger into the flab of my belly. Onstage, the music hit a crescendo and a voice sang a long, sustained high note. I felt a brief pinching, satisfying pain that let me know I was alive, that this was real, that I was a body ready to make another body. Then I counted – one, two, three, four – as the medicine released and I quietly exhaled.

After I'd buttoned myself up, I walked through the bright lobby and pushed open the theatre door. I made my way through the sudden blackness, moved quietly down the aisle and sat down, my pulse peckering at my throat. Lucie reached out and took my hand in the dark. She squeezed it. I felt her hand saying, *Don't worry, I'm here.* And I was glad.

༒

On Friday, 4 January 2019, I put on a short, floral orange sundress – the one I often wore on dates. A fiery summer wind blasted in my face when I opened the front door and hurried to the car to drive myself to the fertility clinic.

Only a handful of friends knew that I was here, on this day, attempting to fork the path of my life. In the lift on the way up to the treatment rooms, I took a selfie in the mirrored doors. There was no vanity in this photo. I wasn't planning to post or share it but I needed a witness, an image outside of myself to preserve history. To capture this secret and electrifying feeling – as though I was standing before the open doors of a plane, ready to leap. A photo that showed that precipice, the minutes before my childfree self leapt into my potential next life as a mother.

The waiting room in the clinic was lined with unoccupied chairs; tinny pop played over the speakers. It felt as if the whole city had emptied out and gone to the coast, that I was the only single woman crazy enough to try to get artificially pregnant in early January. I tried to breathe steadily – to meditate into a state of tranquil fecundity.

I sat opposite a nurse and went through a questionnaire to give my consent. She chattered on, overly friendly, but I felt detached from making small talk. Then I stepped into the IVF room; it was cool and clean. Other people were having lazy summer sex to conceive spring babies. But other bodies and sex were very far away from this room.

Kate bounced into the room in blue scrubs. She smiled. 'The sperm looks good.' I imagined the sperm under the microscope, as it writhed furiously in search of an egg. For sperm, it was all about the destination; not the journey.

I lay down and opened my legs and let Kate insert a narrow catheter filled with sperm into my uterus. I felt a cold, electric ache fly up my body. I winced. 'Are you okay?' Kate asked. I nodded. She took my hand and helped me up. 'Hopefully that's it,' she said.

There was no need, she assured me, to lie prone; sperm could fight the pull of gravity on its way forth. But I figured I should get my money's worth, so I embraced superstition and lay in my small car to preserve every last drop. My body seemed to vibrate with possibility. *I did it, I did it, I did it,* I said to myself.

I couldn't get the seat to recline so I wedged my head up against the door, the handbrake under my back, my feet cramped against the passenger side. I lay as still as I could for fifteen minutes. Outside the window in the carpark, I watched as a couple from the maternity hospital carried their sleeping newborn to their car for its first ride home. The parents' eyes looked down at their baby and I imagined they felt the same things that coursed through me: hope, dumbstruck love, worry. Their eyes never lifted once from their baby's face.

Two-Week Wait

In IVF circles, women nod knowingly, wearily, at you when you mention the two-week wait. Or TWW as it's inscribed on the wall of the solo mothers' Facebook group. It was the limbo between embryo transfer, or insemination, and a pregnancy test (or the unwanted arrival of your period).

Over those two weeks, I had to do two more injections to stimulate the ovaries to produce more hormones to make the lining of my uterus cosy and welcoming so that a fertilised egg would stick. The hormones made me feel moody and bloated.

'They're designed to trick your body into thinking it's pregnant,' the nurse explained (and to give an actual pregnancy a better window for success). Which meant that, maddeningly, hope-stokingly, I was experiencing the symptoms of pregnancy.

Inside me, an invisible process was taking place that was out of my control. The sperm *might* have met my egg and started multiplying, becoming a speck. This speck could be taking root in the garden of my womb.

Or the sperm might not have hit its target at all. Or if it did hit its target, for reasons that no one could explain, the egg may have shrugged off the sperm. Then the egg would unceremoniously croak. In which case, my period would start.

Either way I felt strung out and raw. I was in a liminal space that was neither night nor day. I tried to go about my life with a blank face, as though I was not counting the minutes until I could do a pregnancy test.

I went down to a small coastal village to stay with my parents. They had no idea I was in limbo. We had reached an agreed détente around solo motherhood – I didn't mention it and neither did they. I thought that telling them would open myself up to opinion, which I didn't want, especially when everything inside me felt like the overstretched skin of a balloon, poised to pop and deflate into nothingness.

I thought bitterly of the women who had male partners and fell pregnant 'accidentally' – a description that made pregnancy sound like slipping on a banana peel. I envied those women who didn't realise until their period was late that their insides had irrevocably changed. Women who were spared this excruciating uncertainty.

One hot afternoon, my parents and I sat outside in the garden, shaded by an umbrella, eating halves of tart passionfruit. Everyone else had drifted inside except for my dad and our family friend Barb. Barb was seventy, with a gleaming grey bob in a set mushroom. She was an enthusiast for life and conversation who had a way of fixing her eyes on you so you couldn't edge your way out of a chat. We were idly talking about the merits of passionfruit when, without a beat, Barb veered the conversation sideways. 'I think you should foster a child for six months,' she said.

My hackles immediately rose.

'Why?' I asked.

'So that you can see what it's like to do it alone,' Barb said, implying that I didn't know what I was getting myself into.

Her words were like a sharp smack across my face. I hadn't told Barb that I was trying to become a solo parent. I had shared nothing. Barb and my parents had obviously been talking about me. I felt exposed. What whispered judgements had been shared behind my back?

I looked over to my dad. Sensing conflict, he picked up the chopping board stained with passionfruit juice and vanished through the sliding doors. I didn't know how to respond to Barb. I was still reeling from her presumption.

'I think a child who didn't have a father would feel like a failure,' Barb continued.

There it was. I felt a pulsing behind my ears.

'A lot of relationships fail and children end up without a father,' I said, staring straight ahead, unable to look at her, in case I started to cry from fury.

Barb ignored this.

'I think a child without a father would feel an absence,' she said.

'I think a child born into all this,' I gestured at the garden, the spacious beach house, 'with a grandpa and grandma and uncles would have plenty of love. And a world of privilege.' My breath was shallow. I fished around for some more rebuttal, 'It's not like this is a warzone or something.'

Why was I talking about warzones? Why the hell were we talking about a subject that wasn't hers to talk about with me? That I hadn't shared?

'But this would be a child born of luxury,' she said, 'whereas someone in a warzone may not have had a choice. You have a choice.'

Barb raised her eyebrows as if to say, *Gotcha.*

'I know. It's *my* choice.'

Barb ignored the hint and changed tack. 'If I was in your position, I would be desperate to have a child, so I empathise.' Her sympathy felt lacquered over condescension.

She sighed. 'I really feel for you.'

'Thank you,' I said, hating myself for saying it.

I stood up and got out of there as quickly as I could. Out the front of the house, I paced up and down the pebbled road in bare feet and called Sam.

The line was bad and every third word kept cutting out. Hot, furious tears rolled down my cheeks as I recapped the conversation at top speed.

'What a _____,' Sam said

'What?' I yelled.

'A twat,' Sam yelled. 'Twat.'

I started to laugh, wiping away the snot from my face.

'Who is she to tell you how you can and can't have a child?' Sam exclaimed.

'The way she said it, like we're all so desperate and single. So desperate,' I was ranting.

'Desperate times call for desperate measures,' Sam said dryly. 'I would have clocked her. There's nothing wrong with what you're doing. How could something you want so badly be wrong?' she asked.

That night, we were all supposed to go out for dinner. I declined, preferring to stay wrapped up in my wounded pride, shut in my bedroom like a teenager. My parents had betrayed me. Not only that but I could be pregnant. I lay in bed, hopped up on hormone drugs, feverish and wild. I slept fitfully.

Children need a mother and a father, I heard my mother's voice echo in my head. Like my mum, Barb was implying that to pursue motherhood on my own was selfish. It wasn't the first time I'd heard comments that solo motherhood was selfish but now, in the hormonal sea of fertility treatment, the assumption felt like a hand yanking me under the surface. A warning. If I got pregnant, what was to come?

Then again, as Sam had said, how could something I wanted so badly be wrong? Her words comforted me. But was I wrong? Was I misguided? I knew that an absence of a parent in a child's life could lead to complicated feelings. But this so-called *lack* was outlined and sharpened by the pervasive idea of the correct family: one man, one woman and their genetic children.

People like Barb still believed in this 1950s picture despite the myriad of families – same-sex couples with kids, divorced or separated single parents, grandparents raising grandchildren and adopted children. And absent fathers were a trope for a reason: because there were plenty of shitty dads out there. I was doing my future kid a favour by not foisting one of those on their life, wasn't I?

At sunset, I marched up the sand dunes alone, dragging the dead weight of my anger past the gnarled melaleuca trees. I rounded the bend to the top of the hill and a bench where you could watch the sweep of surf below.

From the top of the dunes, the beach curved around to a lighthouse. A pair of small figures walked along the shoreline towards the flashing light. The shush of surf was a shell to my ear; and a symphony of vastness. My anger shrunk and rippled away; my life now a grain of sand.

The next day, as Barb was leaving, she leant over the couch where I was sitting and fixed me in her gaze. 'I think I offended you. I'm sorry. We should support and celebrate you like anyone else having a baby.'

Again, I was flummoxed, not from anger but at her willingness to apologise. In my family, no one admitted being wrong. Our family's way was to get over an insult by pretending it hadn't happened, until the bitterness twisted itself into an ulcer, that will probably kill us before our time.

After Barb had hugged me goodbye, I walked over to the beach for a dip and surveyed the surf. To my left, way out to sea, the green surface puckered as small waves pushed in all directions against each other.

As a teenager my friends and I had got caught in that rip. We were strong swimmers but it had happened without us noticing – suddenly we were whooshed out to sea, towards a stretch of water known as shark alley. A lifesaver, a little man in a yellow and red cap with a rubber dinghy, had beelined out to save us.

Trying to please everyone in my life would be like trying to push my body out directly against that rip. The only way out of a rip was sideways, swimming diagonal to the current – and even then, you had to be a bloody strong swimmer.

I looked around at the beach, where seagulls were dotted between families and teenagers in groups and couples. I looked down to my abdomen, which told me nothing. I had dived willingly into this part of my life and it was rough out here. There was no man coming to save me. Whatever happened, I would have to swim out sideways.

Oh My Goddess

Aphrodite, Oshun, Isis. Each of the cultures around the world had so many fertility deities. I was trying to remember them as I pressed my phone to my ear, pacing the carpark behind my work. I was on hold to the IVF clinic. I was waiting for the results of my pregnancy test.

I stared at a clotted mass of rubbish in the gutter, trying to focus my nerves. The hold music sounded like a Casio version of 'Chariots of Fire' with a manic beat underneath that was making my heart go into overdrive. Every now and then it was interrupted by a recorded voice. 'Thank you for your patience, we'll be with you shortly.'

Mama Ocllo, Bhavani, Brigid. Other cultures had multiple deities that ruled fertility – that's how coveted fertility was. The peoples who believed in them had wisely placed the power to procreate outside their own bodies and into the hands of the fickle gods.

I hadn't prayed to any gods. In our secular world, it felt like a woman's ability to grow and birth a baby represented personal success or failure, despite the workings of our body being out of our control.

The hold music was still stuttering its up-tempo beat. 'Thank you for your patience. We'll be with you –' Not again.

'Hi Alexandra, are you there?'

'Yes, yes, I'm here,' I said. *Tell me, tell me now.*

'Okay …' The nurse paused. She was killing me slowly.

'Your bloods were a low positive,' she almost mumble-slipped the word *low* as though she'd said it by mistake. 'Your hCG is high but not high enough.'

'What does that mean?' I asked, frantic.

'You'll have to repeat the test. But you can be cautiously optimistic. Most likely you're pregnant.'

Everything around me disappeared. Blink. Breathe. An anchor hooked my heart and yanked it upwards then let it go like a boulder falling through my chest.

I managed to take a breath. The whole world flooded back in.

'You'll need to take another blood test on the weekend,' the nurse was saying, 'and then you can have the results on Monday.'

It was Thursday. I would have to wait three whole days.

I walked up the steps to my office, my hands trembling. I went into the bathrooms and locked myself in a cramped room with a shower cubicle. Other than the toilet, it was the only private place to be. I didn't know whether I was terrified or overjoyed – all I could register was a kind of shock. I began to cry – emotion quickly rising to the surface then receding so that my face was dry, my hands still shaking.

This was not how I thought the story would go. I'd assumed that, like so many other women I knew, I'd be felled by disappointment. That my naïve optimism that I could get pregnant would be dashed. That, like so many other areas of my life – in love and my career – I would encounter setbacks and obstacles to getting what I wanted. It was inconceivable that I had simply conceived. I felt guilty that I may have beaten the odds.

Fertility was cruel and capricious. We believed we had power over our bodies but fertility toyed with us. My possible pregnancy was a matter of dumb, grateful, maddening luck.

You might be reading this and thinking, how dare she get pregnant? You're right. I can't even begin to fathom the fury and grief of all the women who wanted to get pregnant but couldn't, who got pregnant then miscarried, who tried again and again. It wasn't, it isn't, fair.

Mara had had many failures before success. Should I tell her or wait?

I needed to place the startling news outside of myself before it drove me mad. I sent Mara a message that my IUI had maybe, possibly worked?

Right now, you're pregnant. Hold onto that, she wrote. *I'm so excited for you.*

Two days later, on Saturday, I got up extra early and went to the local medical centre. I sat waiting in the Communist grey chairs for another blood test. Around me sat the cheerful elderly – facing all the aches and iniquities of aging that came towards the end of one's life. While inside me, a speck was perhaps just beginning its existence.

All weekend, I kept intoning the phrase, *Trust what you can't see* in a spiritual loop while I waited. *Trust what you can't see.* I waited and I wanted. I so badly wanted that the waiting was unbearable.

On Monday, I got the call. I was officially pregnant. Pure elation rushed through me. It had worked. My gods and goddesses, it had worked.

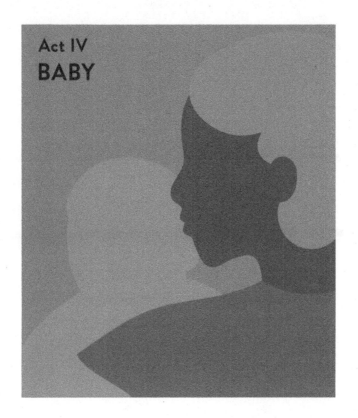

Act IV
BABY

Inconceivable

On-screen a minute blur quivered in rapid motion: a heartbeat. Kate was doing my seven-week scan. 'Look at that,' she said, in a quiet voice I'd never heard her use before. 'Isn't that incredible?' I looked at the screen. I looked at Kate. I didn't feel anything. What was wrong with me? I couldn't translate what was on-screen to what was happening inside me. My body, from the outside, revealed nothing.

As I left, she said, 'Good luck.' I was confused, then I realised, she was sending us forth into the world. Her job, if all went well, was done – from now on my care would be ferried between a GP and the public hospital midwives and obstetricians. 'Make sure you send us pictures and come visit,' Kate called to me as I left her rooms. It took me a few seconds to understand that she meant pictures of the baby. A visit with the baby. The baby. That jittering speck on-screen was a baby. My baby.

Every time my mind went to the pregnancy, it was knifed by a hot, sharp point of disbelief. *I'm pregnant*, I thought, then I immediately cancelled the thought. It was the same way I had felt years earlier when Lucie had called to tell me that our friend had been killed while riding her motorbike. 'No, no,' I'd kept saying to Lucie on the phone, 'that can't be right.' My mind refused it.

Except that this was not death, it was life. It was not grief, it was disbelief. To face it was to stare into the blinding diamond-glitter of creation: breathtaking and frightening.

There were women in the weeks ahead who would quietly fall away from my life and stop speaking to me for months and sometimes years. I didn't blame them. The wonder of what I'd experienced, the stupid one-strike luck of it was too much, it stabbed at something fundamental: at their own agony of missed conceptions. I felt guilty for my luck. I didn't know how to speak about it with them nor they with me. What could I say to comfort them when my body was a herald of their grief?

I called Sam and she crowed with delight. 'I'm brimming with joy. I'm overflowing with joy,' she said. Her words unlocked a feeling that I realised was underneath the terror: pure exhilaration. I was going to have a baby. I couldn't yet let myself fall into the pleasure of getting what I had wanted though. I felt like it might jinx everything, that the cells inside me would stop multiplying.

Sam was easy to tell. But I couldn't picture my mother's reaction. Recently I had stood in her kitchen making a salad. 'You're cutting the tomatoes wrong,' Mum said. 'You should be cutting them the other way.' If I was capable of such a small slip-up with a knife then what would be her reaction to the way I was slicing open the space-time continuum to create a human? So I burrowed into silence and said nothing.

Not only that. Nothing was given or promised. A pregnancy was not a living baby on earth. The two-week wait to find out if I was pregnant was infinitesimal compared to the nine months that stretched ahead of me, during which any number of things could go wrong. First, I had to make it to the twelve-week mark –

when the chance of miscarriage substantially dropped. That was reason enough to wait before I told my parents.

∽ⱷ∾

In those early weeks of my pregnancy, my body was a mask. There were no signs that I was pregnant. I felt bursts of an effervescent, bubbling-over wonder followed by worry.

Then everything shifted. At the seven-week mark, I became perpetually queasy, with the constant hungover sensation of morning, midday and afternoon sickness. There was a lead-in-my-veins exhaustion. I was sleepwalking through a Melbourne heatwave. The shock of what I had done started to subside as smells grew unbearable: a stranger's sweat on the tram, bolognaise bubbling on the stove, the tang of a rubbish truck passing on the street. Parallel to my physical afflictions ran relief because this was proof that I was pregnant; that the imperceptible was taking place inside of me.

I visited my parents and sat by their pool, dangling my legs in the water. I was floating, while inside my womb, the zygote floated in me. I wondered if it would soon begin to form a womb and ovaries. Inside I watched my parents talking silently behind the glass in the air-conditioned cool. They glanced at me. Did they know? Had they guessed?

I went inside and saw my brother Nick's face flashing up on my phone. My parents were in the kitchen, in earshot. 'How's it going? Pregnant yet?' he asked through the phone.

'Mmhm,' I said.

He let out a guffaw. 'Are you serious?'

'Yep,' I tried to keep my voice even, as though I was confirming the weather.

I could hear him telling Ellen in the background and her exclaiming with delight.

'Congratulations,' he said, still in disbelief. I hung up and looked up at my parents who hadn't noticed a thing. I needed to tell them, the secret was making me itchy.

Back at my place, Lucie was lying on the couch, scrolling on her phone, distracted when I told her. She looked up sharply. 'Really?' she said. 'Really!' She quickly corrected herself. 'I can't believe it. I mean congratulations, that's great.' I couldn't quite tell what she felt. Telling her, my single, childfree friend felt like prodding at something tender, at an unspoken question: *Will this change things between us?*

Each day there was a pounding in my brain that was making work impossible. I was flying to New York in a few months for the ill-timed rehearsals and production of my Off Broadway musical. I'd agreed to the production last year, not quite believing I'd get pregnant so quickly. Now I was receiving insistent emails from the director and the producer requesting the latest, finished draft. I hadn't told them I was pregnant yet.

Instead of writing, I wandered through the heat, stupefied. I ate, napped then felt the sickness rise and ate, napped and so on.

I went to the bar where my brother Tom worked. It was quiet and Tom was leaning on the bar, hunched over, looking into his phone. He saw me and straightened up. I ordered a soda water and sat on a stool. He picked up a clean glass and started filling it with post-mix.

'How's it going?' he asked.

'Well, I'm pregnant.' I grinned at him.

'What!' he put the glass down and I saw the good shock of it hit him, his mouth widened into a beam.

'That's incredible. That's amazing. I'm so happy for you. I'm so, so happy for you.' He came out from behind the bar and hugged me. His pure delight filled me up. I didn't realise it was possible to hand someone a secret and feel this much goodness.

'It makes sense,' he said, 'because my horoscope said that in my late twenties, I would be a hero, possibly to a child.' He laughed and dipped his head forward in his self-deprecating way.

'You can be my child's hero,' I said. 'I fully endorse that. I'm sure you'll be a cool uncle.'

'Have you told Mum and Dad?'

'Not yet, I was going to wait till twelve weeks but it's killing me. I'm going to tell them at dinner next week,' I said.

'Oh God. I might have to get drunk from second-hand anxiety.' Tom ducked back behind the bar where a customer was waiting. 'Sorry, mate, what can I get you?' he asked.

I watched Tom effortlessly flip the tap and pour a beer, which looked strangely unappetising. My nausea had made alcohol seem wretched.

'What do you think Mum and Dad will say?' I asked, watching the golden liquid fill the glass.

'I have no idea, could go so many ways with Mum, you just never know. I mean I'm sure they'll be nice ...' He put down the beer and left a pause for doubt to creep in.

'Maybe you could film their reaction?' I asked.

The idea of filming my parents' reaction landed on me with fervour. As if filming them could protect me from harm; provide me with a capsule for later if things went awry.

'Sure, just give me a signal,' Tom said.

'Can I just give you like a really intense crazy eyebrow?' I asked.

'More crazy than usual?'

'Way more crazy.'

Over the next week, I wrote endless to-do lists: Kegels and writing and packing and buying cheap maternity wear, and taxes and repotting plants. I spent hours hunched over a grant application for the musical at my computer, eating ginger candies to try to stave off the nausea. I scrolled through rental apartments online.

My share house was disbanding and it was time to find somewhere for the baby and me to live, on our own. I toured through apartments on the other side of town – across the river. But despite my panic at finding somewhere to live, I barely lasted one seasick afternoon. Instead, I slept on Lucie's bed, in the stifling dark, and tried to block out all the things I couldn't finish. Lucie came home from work and lay on the bed next to me, comfortably silent.

Lucie's cousin Buddy biked over that evening with groceries and offered to cook me the only thing I could stomach: minestrone. I could have cried with gratitude. There was something so boyish and innocent about the way Buddy unloaded the bright cans of tomatoes onto the countertop and began to chop the carrots.

'Any vibe with Buddy?' Lucie asked me after he'd left. 'He's single now.' She gave me a loaded look.

'I don't have a vibe with Saladas, and I want to put them in my mouth all day,' I said.

Buddy wouldn't be interested in a pregnant woman anyway, I thought. And in my nauseous state, I felt anything but attractive. The possibility of romance, of flirting, of sex, seemed so remote. My body was curving, all hips and ripening breasts and arse. I noticed men staring at my swollen cleavage on the street. But I couldn't imagine touching someone, acting on the swirl of my prickling, pregnant hormones.

Even if I did try at being a pregnant gal about town looking for the pleasure of a hook-up, chances are I'd be looking for love. I'd be looking for a grown-up who would place a firm hand on my belly and stare into my eyes like we were in a telenovela. A man who was on board with all this. And that was too much to hope for. Too giant a longing to pin on any human man.

My sleep and my sanity and energy were more important than seduction. I needed to focus on willing the baby into existence. I downloaded an app which showed a three-dimensional image of a shrimp-like creature floating in the womb at its actual size. The app told me the baby only weighed about four grams. I stared obsessively at the veiny image, with its alien head. Its dinosaur-like spine appeared at one point to have a tail, but it had grown out of that. I knew the photo-real image on-screen was not my baby but some part of me believed it was my baby. *Keep going*, I thought. *You can do it.*

The restaurant where my family was meeting was tucked off Flinders Lane in the city. It was dark and gleaming and Peruvian. As I walked in, I noticed a raw bar of oysters and slabs of pink and white fish draped over confettied ice. If I was in any doubt about telling my parents, the minefield of things I shouldn't eat and drink on the menu would force the truth out.

I was late and my family were all waiting, tucked into a leather booth, already drinking wine. My sister-in-law, Ellen, was there too, she was visiting from Sydney for work and she'd come without my brother Nick. We all kissed hello on the cheek. Ellen squeezed me in a hug as if to say silently, *Congratulations.* She knew I was planning to announce my pregnancy tonight.

'Do you want a drink, darling?' Dad pointed at his glass of pinot.

I shook my head.

Ellen was gesturing with her elegant dancer's hands, regaling my parents with a story about a musical she was working on as the associate director.

I took a sip of water. My heart was ricocheting around in my chest. I contemplated the menu. Every dish seemed to be ceviche. Raw fish, depending on how strict you were, was not recommended for pregnant women.

My family had their heads bowed, murmuring over the menu.

I planned to wait, to give Tom the signal to start filming with his phone but then I opened my mouth.

'Well, I can't eat raw fish because I'm pregnant,' I blurted out.

The whole table let out a cry of wonder. My mum's mouth dropped open like a clown at a carnival arcade. My sister-in-law gasped and threw her arms up in delight at my lack of ceremony. Tom, to everyone else's confusion, was exclaiming, 'The signal, where was the signal?'

My dad leapt up from his seat and hugged me. My mum followed.

'Congratulations, darling,' they were talking over each other.

'It worked the first time,' I said.

'You're just like your mother, very fertile,' my dad joked.

My parents were bright-eyed, shining. The relief. Oh, the sweet relief.

'I hope it's not twins,' Mum said.

'So do I,' I said.

After the table had settled down, I said, 'I thought you knew, that you would have guessed because I haven't been drinking.'

'We had no idea,' Mum said. 'How many weeks are you?'

'Eight weeks,' I said. She hmmm'd but kept a lid on saying anything about it being too soon to tell people.

'I'm not telling everyone, just family and a few friends.'

'I think that's a good idea. Did you ride your bike here?'

I nodded, waiting to be in trouble.

'Your brain gets foggy when you're pregnant. Riding is not safe,' Mum said. 'You can borrow my car while you're pregnant.' Her offer was an invisible line reaching out between us. I was grateful.

My parents' rapture felt like a blessing. Perhaps, I thought, from now on, things between us would be easy.

I didn't know what was to come.

Good Mother

I had made it to twelve weeks and, after cresting that hill, I saw an infinite stretch of winding, climbing paths ahead of me. There were the genetic tests, which I was waiting on the results for. I didn't let my mind wander to what I would do if they revealed something unexpected. There was negotiating a permanent work contract with my job before I told them I was pregnant. There was writing and fundraising for my musical and travelling to New York. There was the question of where I would live. Which is why I was standing in my bedroom surrounded by open boxes and clothes exploding out of bags. I'd given up on trying to find my own apartment until I got back from New York – instead I'd move into another share house for a few months.

Lucie was cheerfully throwing my belongings into boxes and bags with a can-do spirit that I could no longer muster. Despite making it to the end of the first trimester, I still felt constantly ill.

'Where am I going to put all this stuff?' I slumped onto the bed.

'Some of it can go to my new house,' Lucie said as she grabbed a roll of sticky tape and screeched it across a box to seal it up. The sound and the chemical smell of the sticky tape made me shut my eyes and wince.

'Thanks. I don't know what to do with the rest of the bags though.'

'Call your mum. Now.' Lucie was not suffering my whininess.

My mum answered straight away.

'How are you feeling, darling?'

'Ugh. Pretty nauseous but apparently nausea means the baby is intelligent?'

'Well, I'm sure the baby will be intelligent.' I could hear her pleasure at imagining her future grandchild.

'At least I know I'm still pregnant.' I was stalling because I hated asking for favours.

'Mmm.' She was distracted – I could hear it, probably swiping letter tiles into different configurations on Words With Friends. I needed to corral her attention before I lost her.

'So I was wondering if it would be okay if I left a few suitcases at your house while I'm away? Just until I get back from overseas.'

She paused before she spoke. 'It's not really convenient for us,' she said. A coldness had entered her voice.

Lucie raised her eyebrows at me expectantly. I mouthed 'nup' at her. Lucie shook her head.

'It would just be for a few months,' I explained.

'We're getting a lift put in so we're not going to have any space,' Mum said.

A door slammed shut between us.

I didn't point out that my parents had a large house for two people to live in, that they'd hardly notice a suitcase or two. There was no point pushing when Mum had made up her mind.

As I headed towards motherhood, it was becoming clear to me that when I encountered my mother, I never knew which mother

I'd meet. The endlessly generous, loving mother or the mother who found me to be an inconvenience.

Had she always been like this? As a child, my mum had a repertoire of silly faces to entertain us. Tongue poked out, eyes rolled back, she'd use her own hands to mime someone choking her neck to make us all laugh. Or she'd get on all fours, growling, 'I'm the kissing MONSTER!' as she chased us down the hall. We'd run with ecstatic terror until she finally caught us and kissed us loudly on our faces and tummies, as we squirmed and giggled.

We loved her. We feared her. One minute she was the kissing monster, the next minute a monstrousness took hold of her. It wasn't volume or her hands that she used as weapons but her intelligence. 'You're selfish,' she snapped at me as a child, shaming me for wanting and doing childish things.

No, that's not right. My mother loved – *loves* – us with ferocity. My mother bought us puzzles and books and took us to the theatre. She read to us, over and over. She cultivated a life of the mind, a way of looking at the world that made me into a writer.

She had told us stories about her childhood with her own complicated, mentally ill mother. My grandmother had, in a rage, chased my mother around the house with a large carving knife. Until my grandfather intercepted her. I wondered if my mother still saw that knife-glint in her dreams.

My mother who carried the bleeding world: the sick, the poor, the mentally ill, the children. She worked as a GP in a clinic under the housing commission flats where she was devoted to her patients, the Ethiopian and Sudanese and Kenyan refugee mothers and their babies. My mother who was given an OAM for her volunteer work on the board of a mental health organisation. She was always donating money to charities.

My mother at the Melbourne Club – Melbourne's elite club for men that occasionally held events that wives could attend – a club that had a history of exclusion. 'You really need to have more Muslim members,' my mother lectured the head of the club.

My mother who occasionally bit her tongue when her conservative friends castigated the poor for being dole bludgers. Although, in truth, my mother was never much good at biting her tongue. Her friends described her as candid and exact and witty and opinionated and fierce and glamorous and analytical.

My mother who loved a party, loved her friends, loved people – who was endlessly giving and unforgivingly sharp. My mother who told me as a child that I was 'the most beautiful girl in the world'. My mother who said, 'Hello, darling,' in the most tender of voices when she saw me.

My mother who was a hundred mothers in one. Who ruled my father and our house. Who was smarter than all of us. Who I could never live up to.

My mother who comforted me, years ago, when I had been sad in San Francisco. I'd followed Dave there for a few months while he worked on a show. I was rudderless and broke and depressed. Mum wrote and told me about a time she felt similarly lost when she was five months pregnant and what appeared out of that darkness.

Indeed something wonderful did arrive for me at the time I am talking about. It was you. A whole new world opened to me and I had an amazing new person in my life who transformed the world for me. Dad and you and Nick and Tom are the best things that have ever happened to me.

I hadn't completely understood, in my longing to have a baby, that a baby would also make me a mother. What kind of mother would I be? Like all parents, I hoped to fill the blind gaps and wounds that my parents had left. I promised to be different, to always say, *I love you* and *I'm proud of you* and *I believe in you.* But no matter how much I loved my child, I knew I'd fail in some way; that I'd be the source of complicated feelings.

My child who I was sure was a girl. Every day I stared at the app, at the floating creature. The littlest thing. Barely measurable, barely visible, but I felt her to be tenacious already. The will to live was strong. I had a vision of a little girl; fearsome and capable. I was sure that she was forming inside me. Another daughter to continue the lineage of eldest daughters on both sides of my family. How would I mother her? Could my mother tell me how?

Now that I was pregnant, it felt like I needed my mother more than ever. The encouraging mother. But it was my stubborn mother who was refusing to store my belongings. Was it always going to be like this, once I had a baby?

Everything will be okay, said a lulling voice in my head. The moving. The trip. The musical. Finding a home. Giving birth. Everything will be okay, I believed superstitiously, because being single warded off other evils. Surely, I would not be given more challenges: a roofless existence, a theatrical flop Off Broadway, a frail baby kept at the edge of life with tubes and wires. It was as though there were scales of justice measuring my life: on one scale, I stood alone, but this was balanced by the other scale, which held the weight of a healthy baby. This superstitious approach blocked out all the good things I'd been gifted that could tip the balance: my bountiful privilege, my one-shot wonder pregnancy.

A few days later, I sat in the doctor's office waiting for the results of the genetic test. I was testing out a new GP, trying to find the right person for my pregnancy care. The doctor prattled on as she looked through the paperwork to find the results. 'I swam forty laps every day of my pregnancy right up to birth,' she said. 'With twins.' I made a half-hearted sound of being impressed.

'This says you went through Melbourne IVF?'

'I was inseminated,' I said. 'My baby is donor conceived.'

'Ahh. Quite an adventure you've set yourself,' the doctor said in a jaunty tone that was concealing either pity or disapproval. She was not the right doctor. I needed to call Mum, who would be able to recommend a good GP. My mother, who always had the answers to anything medical.

'Okay, what have we got here?' The doctor finally found the right piece of paper. 'Everything looks good, no abnormalities on the genetic tests.'

I exhaled.

'Do you want to know the gender?'

I nodded.

'You're having a boy,' she said.

'Really?' I asked. 'Really?' I was stunned.

After the appointment, I called my dad.

'Hi, darling, how are you?' his voice was garbled through the speaker phone of his car.

'Good ... So, I'm just calling to tell you you're going to have a grandson ... I'm having a boy.'

'A boy! Terrific,' he exclaimed. I know he would have been just as thrilled with a girl.

'Mum and I are going to be even more outnumbered by testosterone.'

'A boy. That's great news.'

I could hear the pleasure in Dad's voice. His joy shot through me and became my own.

I took comfort in the dad-ness of my dad: solid and reliable and gruff, a man who expressed love through acts of service. My dad who brought my mum a cup of tea every morning, who was always willing to drive us to the airport and to drill or putty a wall for me. I knew that as a daughter I was less hard on him than I was on my mother. How often daughters cut their fathers the slack that their mothers most deserve. I sensed that Dad would be there, willingly, for my son, no matter what.

My son. A boy. While I knew that gender didn't matter, I sensed a shift. A new reality. A firstborn boy to interrupt the thorny legacy of mothers and daughters.

Immaculate

I'd become pregnant without having sex. Yet my pregnancy was more salacious than a one-night stand. How would I tell people?

At my first intake appointment at thirteen weeks, at the Royal Women's Hospital, the young midwife sitting opposite me had barely concealed her eagerness when she found out I'd conceived with donor sperm. 'Can I ask you a personal question?' she leant forward. I glanced out the window at the anodyne medical high-rises, and thought, *Please don't*. But she continued, conspiratorial: 'Did you just want to have a baby?'

The midwife was looking at me. *Did I just want to have a baby?* 'Yes,' I answered, choosing the simplest route, because the one to finding my way here had been anything but.

Mara had announced her own pregnancy on Facebook as her *Immaculate Scientific Conception*. Another solo mum I knew had gathered her entire Indian family and friends at a local hall for a party and stood up to make the announcement over a microphone. The crowd had applauded.

I hadn't revealed my pregnancy publicly yet. Partly because I was in the midst of negotiating a contract for permanent employment. Partly because I wasn't sure how to announce it. My immaculate scientific conception was still a secret.

I may have conceived using science but as my body swelled, and the nausea abated, I felt like flesh and blood again. My nerve endings pulsed with the rush of extra plasma that a pregnant woman's heart pumps through her body. When I walked down the street, it felt like a thousand radiating antennae strained upwards from my skin, wanting to be touched.

Buddy and I had been texting. Harmless texts where he offered to pick up groceries or drive me to my studio. There was a sturdy, benign quality to our friendship. I had a sense that I could rely on him, no matter what. He had invited me around to watch *The Fugitive* at his flat in a few nights' time. Our friendship usually existed in Lucie's shared orbit. I had never been to his apartment on my own. Surely, there wasn't another motive to his invitation? I was leaving town soon to go to New York for two months for my musical. I was also pregnant. Now wasn't a good time to start something.

I had more pressing problems. I still hadn't told the ad agency that I was pregnant. Sixteen weeks pregnant.

Over the past few months, I'd sat at my desk, constantly opening and closing a black metal drawer filled with Saladas. I crunched as quietly as possible, trying to keep my nausea on a leash. I was aware that I was lying, by omission. My much-wanted baby felt like a betrayal of my job. I veered between fuck-it-to-hell self-talk (*I'm happy I'm pregnant! This job wasn't even what I'm born to do. I'm truly a writer, goddamnit. Did Hemingway work for an ad agency? No, he didn't. He would have spat on this job. I spit on this job!*) and anxiety (*You think you can have a baby and it'll all be fine, that you'll be able to come back to work? That they won't somehow fire you or demote you? You need this job so don't fuck it up.*

You're a single mother. You can't afford not to return to work after three months of maternity leave.)

The days were passing, and my waist was noticeably expanding. I had to come clean. I'd finally finalised my contract, which had involved a delicate dance to negotiate unpaid leave to go to New York for my production. I was leaving soon. I could hardly arrive back from New York and walk into work with a mound at my middle: *Ta da, I'm six months pregnant!*

But there was something else stopping me from announcing my pregnancy. It was one thing for my close friends and family to know. The reaction from those near to me had been a cascade of loveliness – with the occasional hiccup of confusion (*Is this good news?* a male friend texted me. *Do I know the father?*) But telling work was different. My colleagues and I were friendly but not friends. There was something so public about revealing this part of myself to them.

What assumptions would they make? They knew I was single. *She must have had a one-night stand with a stranger*, they would say.

Did you hear? I imagined them whispering with glee by the espresso machine. *She was SINGLE and so DESPERATE to have a baby that she used a stranger's sperm.* To announce my pregnancy would be a collision of my most private wants – this baby – with the breezy, public self I presented at work.

My public self was careful to present as independent and smart and ambitious – a woman who'd moved ten thousand miles across the globe to be a playwright. But my private self was primal and soft and full of longing. Revealing my pregnancy would unpeel my public self to reveal a vulnerability that I hid in case it stirred the most loathsome thing of all from others: pity. So, I sat at my desk quietly growing and sliding open my drawer full of snacks. Crunch. Crunch. Crunch. And delayed.

♉

I sat in my car outside Buddy's apartment for our movie night. As I stared at the 1970s brick flats where he lived, I knew that when I walked through his front door I would be inviting trouble.

I'd been having odd dreams: one where my baby was born feet first, another where twigs and bark poured from my breasts, making the baby choke. Dreams where there was a man standing in the dark of my bedroom. I could hear him speaking but I couldn't see him. His voice was low and familiar. The invisible man. Was it the sperm donor? Where was he? Why couldn't I find him? Dreams where Buddy and I were kissing but our teeth clunked together awkwardly. I wanted to be touched so badly that I was dreaming it up.

I lay on Buddy's couch, curled on my side, watching the TV, tense with the possibility of where this was going. By the time Harrison Ford was sweaty and thrusting his way out of the wreckage of the prison van, I was stretched across the couch, my feet in Buddy's lap. 'Do you want me to rub your feet?' he asked. Of course, I did. 'Is that okay?' he asked as he steadily kneaded his thumb into my arches. I could feel the tensed parts of my body scatter-drift like petals.

The movie finished. 'If you want, I can massage you lying down, on my bed?' he asked.

My belly was still small enough that I could lie on my stomach. My face was smushed into Buddy's duvet. I inhaled. Tree bark, woody and dense. Cut with detergent. He moved his thumbs beneath the wings of my shoulder blades. Then pressed them gradually upwards. I felt the popcorn flickers of the baby kicking. By the time Buddy was dragging his hands along the base of my neck, my body was evaporating: steam and air.

'That's kind of dangerous,' I said, my voice underwater, facedown.

'What? Why?'

'Touching my neck like that ...'

'Oh really?' he asked in a teasing voice.

'Yeah, that's where the button is that switches off my logical brain,' I garbled into the pillow.

He moved his mouth to my neck and began to kiss along the nape. I turned to face him.

'Kiss me,' I said.

'Not yet.'

He kissed along my neck for an agonisingly long time.

I nuzzled my mouth towards him. My lips briefly met something soft, but he played coy, pulling his mouth back. I tried again. And then our mouths fitted in a way that was far better than a bad dream. I heard myself sigh into his mouth.

I ran my hand along his wrist which was circled by the thick black line of a tattoo. I pulled his t-shirt over his head. His chest was hard and smooth apart from a few stray wisps of hair that curled in opposite directions. I felt self-conscious about revealing my pregnant body. I was only sixteen weeks – a small bump – but would he still want me even though I was becoming a mother?

When he pulled up my dress and touched my bare skin with his hands, everything went static. I became hazy, like a shimmer of sea on the horizon. *If sex was supposedly for reproduction, then why were pregnant women so horny?* And after that, I was beyond thought, my legs straddling his legs, his thumbs digging into my hips, riding wave upon wave of pleasure.

Afterwards, I lay with my head in the crook of Buddy's neck, his arm circling me.

'Do you want to feel the kicks?' I asked.

'Sure,' he said.

I took his hand and placed it on the centre of myself.

The baby let out a tiny series of jabs.

'Ahhh.' Buddy's face opened.

The next morning, I left his apartment early for work. I felt high on touch, and exhausted and bewildered. What was I doing? I was single and pregnant. This made no sense. But I could feel that delicious, addictive thrum of attraction magnetising me towards someone new. I shook myself out of the stupor: I was leaving soon. Buddy was young. Buddy was just a friend – it had simply been a one-night thing.

A few days later, Buddy texted to tell me that he'd told his best guy friend that he'd slept with a pregnant woman. *So you had a threesome*, his friend joked. I rolled my eyes.

I minded and I didn't mind. I wanted to be an exotic object of pregnant wonder, but I also wanted to be an ordinary woman that a man would want. I wanted to be my former un-pregnant self and my current self. I was trying to reconcile the fact of my singleness with the growing fact of motherhood. It seemed impossible. Could I be pregnant and still date? Would a man really want a woman who was pregnant with a stranger's sperm?

Buddy and I were old friends and he didn't seem put off by my pregnancy. This was a man who made me minestrone. A man who was sweet and available. A man who was a good kisser. We hadn't talked about the future. But now that sex had come into the equation, I was addled.

Was Buddy the Magical Final Man that I was supposed to meet all along? In the future, I would tell people the story: *I was pregnant, with a stranger's sperm and that's when he appeared. My old friend. Turned out he was the love of my life. The future father of my unborn child.*

Buddy would legitimise my entire pregnancy, adding an air of authoritative maleness to the proceedings. Was that what I longed for? To be like the women in my pregnancy yoga class who were always peppering their conversation with 'my husband' and 'my partner'. Did I just want legitimacy or did I truly think that Buddy and I would fall in love?

No. It was ridiculous. I was being a fantasist. The hormones had got to me.

⚭

I slid the door of the conference room shut and sat down opposite my boss, tall and stooped with a relaxed demeanour and Oscar Wilde hair. I couldn't wait any longer. I felt as though someone had placed a vibrating tuning fork to my skull; a high note rang along the tendons of my neck. I placed a steadying hand on my son under the table. I had nothing to be ashamed of. I took a long inhale then let my breath expel the words I'd been holding in.

'So, I wanted to tell you that I'm pregnant,' I said.

'Congratulations,' he smiled as he tucked his hair behind his ears. He was studied in the art of professional reactions; he didn't pry. 'I thought something was going on when you tried to negotiate paid maternity leave.' We both laughed. I was grateful that he was gracious and unflappable.

'When will you announce it?' I asked.

'Whenever you want.'

I knew that his colleague, Trev, would do a public announcement, that was how things were done. I didn't think to question it.

'Today if possible. Let's just get it out of the way,' I said.

Now the fate of my pregnancy announcement was in Trev's somewhat unpredictable hands. The day dragged; time was like molasses and my nerves were being stretched along its sticky, never-ending drip. Finally, it was 5 pm. A restless end-of-week energy hung in the air as Trev stood up to address us. Everyone wanted him to stop speaking so they could escape into the weekend.

'Well it's a real rollercoaster of news this week,' Trev said.

Then he turned to me. 'Are you sure you want me to say this?'

I blinked, thrown. This did not bode well. He was treating my news as something that shouldn't be spoken. There was a grin on Trev's face, like a naughty schoolboy. I nodded at him.

'Well, um, I'm not really sure of the details,' he chuckled, building up to a punchline.

'But Ally's pregnant …?'

The room let out some stilted applause amid stray giggles.

'It's not his baby!' I called out.

Everyone exhaled with laughter. My face held a rictus smile. Then my youngest colleague, an English rose with sleek blonde hair, walked over to me.

'Congratulations, that's such fantastic news.' She beamed at me. I could have kissed her for her kindness. That, I thought, is how you react to a pregnancy announcement.

Afterwards, I made my way down the hallway but Trev appeared in my path.

'So … do you have a boyfriend?' he asked.

This was it. What I'd been dreading. The assumptions. The questions. The judgement. I smiled brightly and looked him dead in the eye. 'Nope. I used a sperm donor, through an IVF clinic.'

Later, most of my colleagues offered sincere and unquestioning statements of congratulations. But I still found myself rushing to explain. 'I used a sperm donor!' Why did I have to say that? I didn't owe them any explanation. But here I was trying to cloak my pregnancy in propriety. I was furious at myself, at Trev, at how rattled I felt.

When I got home, I sat dead eyed, slumped in my bed, and stared for a long time at the wall. I felt like someone had peeled my skin like a lychee, then sucked at my innards and spat me out.

⚭

Lucie and I were sitting in the ultrasound waiting room at the Women's Hospital in a long line of empty yellow chairs. Next week I would be in New York, so my GP had arranged for an early scan, at nineteen weeks instead of the usual twenty-plus weeks.

A pregnant woman sat opposite us with her male partner, silent.

'So what's happening with Buddy?' Lucie whispered, leaning into me.

'What do you want to know?' I whispered back.

'I mean, don't tell me because he's my cousin and I don't want to know but also tell me everything,' she said. We both let out a low, hissing giggle. It felt inappropriate to be talking about this in a waiting room, where most people were already ensconced in domesticity and foreverness.

I kept my voice low. 'I mean, Buddy and I are friends. And I'm leaving soon. I don't think it's going anywhere.'

'You never know.' Lucie stared at me. 'Imagine if this was it, after going through all this to have a baby on your own ...' It was as though Lucie had read my mind.

Lucie's voice rose to normal volume. 'And then Buddy becomes your baby daddy.'

The pregnant woman opposite glanced up at us. Lucie clapped her hand over her mouth and started laughing. I dropped my face in my hands, performing my mortification for Lucie.

Thankfully, the sonographer, who looked to be in his twenties, with a checked shirt and a receding hairline, called out, 'Alexandra?'

In the ultrasound room, we sat in the semi-dark. The sonographer seemed nervous, as he squirted the gel onto my stomach. He pushed the monitor onto my belly. On-screen in front of me, the perfect snub-nosed profile of the baby's head appeared. 'Ohhhh,' Lucie cried out. She pulled out her phone and started to film the screen. Then turned the phone to me and started snapping photos.

'It must be incredible getting to do this all day,' said Lucie to the sonographer. She was using her flirty voice.

'You can't take photos,' the sonographer said.

Lucie gave me a cheeky, wide-eyed look and put her phone away. The sonographer moved the wand across my skin. His quiet was disconcerting.

'How's everything looking?' I asked.

The sonographer was concentrating on drawing little dotted lines along the baby's limbs on-screen.

'Measurements are normal,' he said. 'Placenta is out of the way, which is good,' he said. 'We'll check the heart activity.'

Lucie pulled her phone out and I mouthed at her: *No.* We were about to start giggling again, on the precipice of teenage hysteria. But then the galumphing of the heartbeat came through the speaker. We fell silent. We stared at each other. The wonder of it. My boy.

The sonographer took the monitor away and the heartbeat vanished. 'Can I hear it again?' I asked.

⚇

A few days later, Buddy was driving me to the airport. We hadn't seen each other since our night together weeks earlier. As the grey ribbon of highway slipped past, I felt Melbourne tugging at my body.

But I was heading to New York, where it was almost summer. I had a production to get through. A baby to grow. I needed to be sensible. I had it all rehearsed. I would not fall into a going-nowhere romance while I was pregnant. I was weary and wary of love, and Buddy, like Dave, was younger than me. A man-boy still growing into existence.

'I think it's best if we don't get strung out, send messages for months and create something between us that isn't there while I'm away,' I said.

'I agree,' he said. A little too quickly.

I sat silently as the buildings were replaced by blanched winter grass.

On the kerb at the airport, amid the hurry of cars ejecting travellers and suitcases, I hugged Buddy tightly. Then I kissed him firmly on the mouth and walked away.

Off Broadway, Baby

For actors to have stepped onstage for an Off Broadway musical, for the lights to dip to black and rise, for the opening chords to play, for that first harmony to be sung required a series of steps. Those steps were invisible to an audience member sitting in the cabaret-style theatre, shovelling a shoestring fry into their mouth and swallowing it down with chardonnay on opening night.

For the composer and I it had started eight years earlier, in 2011, when we had met in a Brooklyn café as strangers – two Australian women trying to be artists in New York. We ate breakfast burritos and talked about how we liked each other's work. We decided that maybe, perhaps, we could write something together? No big deal.

Then we went away and sent each other scraps of ideas. I wrote some terrible poetry and she rewrote my words into perfect songs. We decided to throw a night of short works up in a friend's loft in Brooklyn. We wrote a ten-minute musical, found a mate to direct it and some wildly talented actors to work for free. Our friends sat on cushions on the floor and drank cheap red wine and applauded.

Then there were the applications: the residencies, the grants, the fellowships. We took the musical west to a residency in Wyoming where the earth looked like the moon, meerkats roamed and ancient crop circles could be traced on the hills. Then to upstate New York where we were put up in an idyllic house hidden along a dirt road for a week.

We spent minutes and hours and days and years in rooms over pages and a piano throwing ideas back and forth. We killed off characters, we stripped away the premise and wrote another, we kept our protagonist.

There were rewrites. Then readings. Developments where actors stood with scripts in hand and performed to a half-empty theatre with dust balls under the seats. There was the composer's IVF treatment. There were the arguments. The years where we were on hiatus, barely speaking. The reunion. More rewrites. The interest from theatres. The rejections. The worry. Eventually, the babies – hers and now mine in utero. There was a musical competition in Sydney where a greying man on the panel asked us if we'd ever bothered to read Gershwin's or Sondheim's work. 'These are not good lyrics,' he declared pointing to the stage, to what we women had made.

And now, eight years later, we had been offered a production at Joe's Pub at The Public Theater. The Public was a New York institution, a large Victorian red brick and stone building with arched windows looming over Lafayette, downtown. It was where *Hair* and *Hamilton* had started. We were ecstatic. Every hour, every argument, every chord, every minute hunched over a desk, every scrap of fundraising, every hope and disappointment had led to this.

On the first morning of rehearsals, still jet-lagged, I walked to the train station from my friend's house where I was staying in New Jersey. I passed the gabled suburban houses in her affluent suburb of Maplewood where progressive Brooklynites fled when they had babies. The chimneys and porches were quiet, the shady streets curled around in soothing loops. Everything was still but the daylight was assaulting me, popping like fireworks behind my eyelids. The sparks trailed down to my stomach and lurched suddenly. I turned to an orderly garden bed of succulents and vomited. I sat down on a rock at the front of the garden and wiped my mouth. A woman appeared from the house opposite with her dog and they both stared at me. I was out of place. No one walked in New Jersey. No one vomited into the manicured garden beds.

I yelled across the street to her: 'I'm pregnant.'

Her face softened; motherhood had saved me. 'Was it the prenatal vitamins? Every time I took those I'd throw up,' she shouted back. I smiled and nodded, too exhausted to tell her that it was not the prenatal vitamins. It was that I had subjected my pregnant body to twenty hours in a metal tube that flew through the sky and deposited me in a place where it was now daylight instead of night. It was my stupid ambition that had led me back to New York, to the place that I'd escaped from three years ago, to where all the ghosts of my past lived. It was that I was trying to have it all: to be a solo mother and a playwright. It was that I was exhausted and terrified and soon to be broke. It wasn't the prenatal vitamins; it was that I was a fool. What was I doing here? If anything went wrong with the baby, I knew I'd blame myself.

I stood and shuffled back to my friend's house. I would not be going to rehearsals today.

☙

In 2012, I was sitting on a bus travelling down Fifth Avenue, past Central Park. It was early summer and I was in love with a man I'd just met. His name was Dave. The New York sky was an aching blue and the sunlight was dappled by the bowers of Central Park, refracting through the bus in flashes of green. I took out my journal and started to write some lyrics.

The city is starving me slowly
But I can't help loving the sky

It was now 2019 and I was sitting in a black-box rehearsal room with stacks of chairs in the corners, pages of scripts in piles on the ground and actors, long limbed and beautiful, slouching against the walls. The composer was sitting behind me breastfeeding her five-month-old who suckled contentedly through all the noise and clatter of rehearsals. In front of the table where the director and I sat, a young red-headed actress, her curls falling into her eyes, was playing chords on a keyboard. She opened her mouth to sing.

The city is starving me slowly
But I can't help loving the sky

Her voice was crystal and grit swooping upwards. I wanted to cry. I cradled my stomach.

The baby hadn't fluttered that morning. It made me nervous when he was still and silent – it was hard to trust that he was in there just floating in the serenity of the amniotic fluid. But as the drums started, he tapped a beat with his feet against his confinement, pushing at my skin.

In the window of the subway on the way home, I kept catching glimpses of the person I saw myself as in New York. The woman I was when I lived here three years ago. A woman who was loved and safe, who went home each day to an American man. In the glass, I saw flickers of the curve of my belly and then that woman was gone. No one offered me a seat on the train. New York hadn't changed but I had.

As the train rattled above ground, I took out my phone and texted Buddy. I'd promised myself that I wouldn't contact him but I'd cracked after a few days away and sent a mildly flirtatious opening. He'd provided a welcome distraction from the worry about the show, the worry about the baby. Now we were texting every day.

The next day, I waddled through early summer up Broadway from Houston to rehearsal. The director was blocking the show at lightning speed. We had three weeks to rehearse the entire musical. The show was about a '90s rock band called Triplight who had disappeared twenty years ago without a trace. Their lead singer, Willow, had reappeared to reveal the story of what had happened, while the ghosts of her former bandmates accompanied her onstage.

We were in our second week and it was clear that things were not going well. The music charts – which notated the chords so the actors and musicians could learn the songs – were in disarray. We were falling behind schedule. The atmosphere in the rehearsal room was as taut as a violin string.

To make matters worse, I had shilled this show to friends and friends of friends and family friends to get them to donate to our fundraising campaign. Our grant application had failed, so I essentially begged to fund the show. I brazenly emailed all my parents' friends in Melbourne and asked them to contribute even though they'd never get a chance to see the show. Thankfully, they had happily donated – no doubt spurred on by the plaintive picture of my solo pregnancy. But their support only made the stakes higher.

I was in New York. I was pregnant. I was having an Off Broadway debut. The collision of all my ambitions had arrived at this moment. But what if it was a failure?

It was live theatre so there was always the possibility that something could go wrong. What if the actors forgot their lines onstage? What if *The New York Times* called the show a *spectacular mess*? What if the audience walked out and I keeled over and died from the shame? *We had to carry out her pregnant dead body*, people who had witnessed it would say. *I mean the show was bad but at least we got a* show, *you know what I mean?* they would snicker.

I kept telling myself that it didn't matter because, at the end of this, in a few months' time I would have a baby. A person I would love above all else.

I wanted to be here and I didn't want to be here. I had no home yet in Melbourne for the baby. I was halfway across the world, alone and pregnant. Each day I stayed, I was losing money that I should have been saving for maternity leave. I wanted to be a playwright who worked in New York; and I wanted to be a mother. It was becoming clear to me now that I was pregnant that each of my wants would continue to orbit and eclipse the other. An endless circle: motherhood and ambition, ambition and motherhood.

Meanwhile time flew forward towards the two deadlines: the opening night and the birth. There was no way back.

Please Forgive Me

My parents arrived just before opening night and generously put me up in a hotel where they were staying. I had been lugging my suitcase to different friends' places but my body could no longer drag my bags across the city and I was relieved to be in a place with crisp, clean sheets, a bath and the comfort of my parents down the hall.

The morning after they arrived, we ate breakfast together in the staid hotel rooms looking out to Fifth Avenue. The room was quiet but for a waitress carrying a rattling tray with a pot of dishwater American tea. After she'd put it down on the table and left, my mum glanced up at me.

'So if you make a profit, do you pay back all the donors?' she asked.

I slathered some more butter on my toast. 'We're just going to cover costs. Barely. Even if the show is sold out.'

I didn't look at her because the spectre of money haunted me: whether we would cover costs for the show, whether I could survive this trip and single motherhood.

'Do you get paid?' asked Dad. Dad always wanted to know if I was getting paid.

'Yeah, but it'll only really cover the cost of my flight.' I shrugged.

My parents took it in; my life in the theatre was bewildering to them. I'd so often presented my triumphs to them like a child leaping up and down for attention. *Look at me! Look at my fellowship or show or residency!* And then invariably been disappointed with their response, which was never as enthused as I wanted. But the profession I'd chosen was foreign to them – if it had been a medical fellowship or residency, they would have been able to comprehend my excitement. They tried their best. They never said, *Why on earth are you pouring everything into an artistic life of penury?* Instead, touchingly, they'd flown across the globe to see the musical.

To prepare my body for the marathon of birth, I decided to take a long walk downtown to the theatre for the tech rehearsals. The sky was a brilliant blue. People streamed across the street at Union Square, over the smoking manholes. I was only a few blocks away from the theatre when I felt a sharp twinge in my pelvis. I shuffled the rest of the way there through throbbing pain. My dad had been saying to me since he arrived, 'You're overdoing it.' I swore at myself silently. He was probably right.

Everyone was sitting in the tense, half dark of the theatre ready to run through the show. The producer was pale, her face taut. The director's face was stony. I sat at the back in a booth. The actors were standing in their positions for the start of the show, waiting for the lights to rise. 'Okay, when you're ready,' the director called out. The opening sound cue blared; it was an indecipherable squawk of drums and piano. An actor started to sing but his mike cut out. Not one of the actors stepped into their lights. Now in the second trimester, my nausea had abated, but as I sat there watching the mess unfold, I felt queasy.

In the afternoon, I went to see my old doctor in Brooklyn. I walked past the ghosts of my past self: on the corner where Dave and I had lived, at the bistro where we ate together and by the subway steps where we kissed goodbye in the mornings.

The doctor opened the door and beamed at me. 'Congratulations!' she said. She got me to lie down on the table. She didn't have a Doppler – the machine that detected a baby's heartbeat – but she offered to try to find it with her stethoscope. As I lay there she put the cold stethoscope on my skin and pushed down on the baby. I slowed my breathing to try to exhale the discomfort of the metal prodding at me.

'How are you feeling?' she asked.

'Good. I mean I'm having trouble walking. My pelvis really hurts but apart from that I feel good. And doing an Off Broadway show while I'm pregnant might kill me but apart from that, I'm fine,' I joked.

She moved the stethoscope again and I waited. 'It's tricky to detect the heartbeat with a stethoscope,' she said. 'I can definitely feel him kicking though.' She smiled.

'He kicks all the time,' I said. 'He's ready to run.' She took the stethoscope out of her ears.

'I can't find it but if you've got regular movements then you should be fine.' I hoped she was right. For now, all my fear was focused on opening night.

In the hotel later, I undressed and stepped into the bath, trying to let the warm water dissolve my disquiet. I picked up my phone to distract myself by texting Buddy.

Hey, finally home. I'm in the bath.
Oh really? Naked I presume.
No, fully clothed in bath. Kidding. Yep. Naked.
Mmmm ... I would like to kiss your soapy neck.
Oh yeah? And what else?

Buddy took me somewhere else by telling me what else.

⚓

I was sitting in the audience next to my parents. It was opening night. The seating was cabaret style – people were dotted around banquets and tables, eating dinner and drinking as waiters tried to sneak past so as not to interrupt the view. I was taking micro sips of wine and holding my breath to silence my walloping heartbeat.

Onstage, the radiant redhead was sitting at the piano. Triangles of blue light illuminated the wall behind her. The redhead was singing those words that I wrote all those years ago on that bus down Fifth Avenue, missing Dave because he was out of town.

The city is starving me slowly
But I can't help loving the sky

I no longer missed him but I wished I could show Dave this. I wished he could see what this creation that I'd spent years of our relationship writing and agonising over had become. He carried the knowledge of the person I was before, in New York. When I lost him, I lost that intimate witness to my life's passage. I wondered what he'd think of all this, of me now, pregnant on my own. Although maybe I wouldn't be alone. After all, there was Buddy. Buddy who was attentive and open and available.

The city is starving me slowly
I'm so weightless, I may just cry

Then the other actors started to harmonise in a discordant way to mimic the sound of the city's car horns. It was so goddamn beautiful that I just died. But it was a good death. It was the kind of death that transcended you to another realm while you went right on being alive.

As the music played, I felt the baby let out small, sharp kicks.

I took my mum's hand and pressed it to the place where my baby's feet were.

'Can you feel that?'

I waited.

'Not really,' she said.

I let go of her hand.

I had hoped that the pregnancy would bring us closer together. She was still somewhere far off, in a place I couldn't always reach. But she had made it here, to New York.

The show had opened. The mikes cut out at times. The actors forgot some lines. But it held together. There had been bursts of pure loveliness. Afterwards, my parents hugged me tightly. 'It was wonderful, darling. Congratulations.' Their praise poured into me and mingled with my relief. I had done it. I had made it. I was a writer; I was a mother.

At breakfast the next day my dad proudly listed all the songs he loved from the show.

'There was only one song I didn't think was as good as all the others. The music was terrific,' he said.

'And so was the dialogue,' Mum said. 'And the actors were wonderful. I don't know how they learn all those songs and play instruments and remember all those lines.'

Each night, I sat in the audience and felt the rapturous and terrible swirl of watching our musical onstage. *I hope you feel this*, I said to the baby. *I hope this is what you remember*, I told him. *I hope you're born with good music rushing through your veins.* I prayed that he hadn't ingested the anxiety and exhaustion of this trip; that I wasn't a bad mother. But now that I was a mother, I'd never not be guilty, so I also said: *Please forgive me.*

Real Love

Buddy was leaning on his car at the airport under Melbourne's smudged June sky. I'd been gone for six weeks. I raised both arms in the air. 'I'm back!' I yelled. Buddy stood, unmoved. He hugged me briefly. No kiss.

The plane trip had been long. It felt like the woman sitting behind me was kickboxing, her jabs landing in the small of my back. I finally turned and asked politely if she could stop. 'It's just there's someone in here kicking me too.' I smiled and pointed at my belly. The woman gave me a death stare. I tried to sleep but there was no comfortable position to exist in.

In the morning, as we'd flown west towards Melbourne, through the window the pink sky of morning had melted into a yellow haze that bathed the strangers around me. I got up and swayed down the aisle to the bathroom. I washed my face and put makeup on to try to fix the sunken skin under my eyes. I sized myself up in the mirror in my grey tracksuit pants with their extendable waist and my baggy, semi-clean t-shirt. I was almost six months pregnant: there was no hiding the schlubby bulk of my body.

When Buddy had last seen me, at nineteen weeks, my pregnancy was just visible. I could still pretend that I was a no-strings-attached girl about town. But now, the weight and the responsibility of what was happening was screamingly evident. Buddy and I had been messaging and talking for my whole trip. *This was becoming something*, I thought. *Something real.* But I worried that Buddy wouldn't want the responsibility that my body so clearly displayed. That despite all of our conversations and messages, he would take one look at me and drive off.

In the car, on that grey drive along the highway into Melbourne, I got a message from Sam with the code to her front door. She had said I could stay with her and Loki, who was now ten months old, for a few days.

'So. Where are we going?' Buddy asked.

'Sam hasn't sent me the code yet,' I lied, staring at my phone as though I was trying to figure out a maths equation.

'You can come to my place for a bit, if you want?'

This was what I'd been angling for.

I looked out the window of the car and tried to reconcile the strange disorientation of travel to avoid the embarrassment of my deception. I'd just been walking through a muggy summer in Park Slope, past the brownstones on Fifth Avenue on a – what day was it? – Sunday. And now it was Wednesday and we were driving past Princes Park in winter – the grass sodden and icy, the air so cold it knifed my skin.

At Buddy's, I showered and put on clean clothes. I felt the leaden sensation of jet lag. I was being dragged underwater by a dead weight. Buddy made me breakfast: moving about the quiet kitchen to assemble homemade muesli. He sat opposite me as I ate. I let myself glance at the hardness of his chest beneath his t-shirt.

I knew I should try to stay awake but I told Buddy that I was tired and I might need to nap.

'Feel free to get into my bed,' he said.

This was my chance. Surely once I was in his bed, he'd make a move.

'I have to go out. I'll be back in about an hour though so nap away,' Buddy said.

I listened as the front door slammed, deflated. Should I go? Had I misread things? I lay in bed calculating how I could get him to make a move without risking more humiliation.

When Buddy arrived home, he came into the bedroom. His nipples were erect from the cold under his grey t-shirt. I lay in his bed, pretending to sleep – my phone softly playing music to keep me awake. He sat down on the edge of the bed, silently tapping on his phone. I waited, body tensed. Then rolled over, opened my eyes and arched my body awake as alluringly as possible in a body that no longer felt alluring.

He was sending emails, he said, as he half-talked to me. He was saying something about the leaked Pentagon papers and Chernobyl and how many times global disaster had been averted. I liked the way his mind turned things over – the riddles he was constantly unpacking. But the more he talked, the more impossible it seemed that he would close the space between us. I wanted more than anything to reach out and touch him.

Buddy yawned and stretched but his body remained as far from me as possible.

Want to get in bed with me? I asked in my mind, but didn't say it.

I cursed myself for my reticence, his reticence, his cluelessness, my desperation.

He got up and went to make tea. I pushed my face into the pillow and tried not to scream as the musician on my phone sang about how he wanted real love, baby. Then a new song clicked over. *That's it*, I thought. *I'm waiting to the end of this song, and then I'm going.*

The musician slid lazily up the guitar chords and whined as Buddy clattered around in the kitchen. I wanted him to sing forever to extend the moment before I had to make a decision.

But the song ended. I sat up quickly. 'Okay, I'm off,' I called out. 'I'm ordering a car.' I pulled the covers up and smoothed the bed. Annoyed. Buddy appeared in the doorway. I avoided his gaze as he lingered, seemingly surprised that I was leaving.

I hunched over my huge middle and tied up my laces. I was disappointed, fire-spittingly furious but my body, my dumb body, still wanted to be touched.

'I'll bring your bags out and wait with you,' he said.

'Thanks,' I mumbled.

At Sam's house, later, I stood in her kitchen surrounded by dishes and crumbs and half-empty baby bottles leaking formula and cried. 'I'm so stupid,' I told her. 'So embarrassed.' How could he possibly want me? I was pregnant. I'd been an idiot to expect something. The way we'd talked while I was away, though. The intimacies we'd shared. 'Surely, that meant something?'

Sam opened her arms and enfolded me in her soft body. She was sympathetic but not surprised. She'd seen it all before and so had I, but I'd been blinded by the hormonal fever of pregnancy.

'You just had an Off Broadway show. In New York.' Sam's voice was muffled and warm on my shoulder. 'And you're pregnant. On your own. You're killing it.' I realised that Buddy hadn't once asked me about New York or the show on the drive home. I had obliterated all my recent achievements in the pursuit of getting him to want me, to love me.

I'd forgotten the endless disappointments of men. The way they danced towards you with possibility and affection then skipped away and hoped you'd disappear rather than face up to what they'd done. The power they wielded, knowingly or unknowingly, which often lacked the attendant grace that the powerful must carry with them.

Later that night, while Sam was out for dinner, I heard Loki crying out in her bedroom. I went and picked him up and lay with him in Sam's bed. He immediately stopped crying. I could feel the warmth of his body breathing next to mine; our living selves a comfort to each other. This was real love.

Shit Shower

It was winter as I expanded into my last uncomfortable trimester. The days were flinty cold but each night I woke from sweating dreams of calamity and chaos. During the day, as I sat at my desk at work, I whirred through the same incalculable sums: which all added up to my being in the red. How could I afford my impending single motherhood? Each weekend I toured through empty, draughty apartments on the south side of the city – trying to imagine my life inside someone's discarded walls. I had moved from Sam's house to another friend's place while I looked for somewhere to live.

Beyond money and where to live and the churning dread around giving birth, the thought that trilled up and down my spine more than anything else now was: what kind of mother would I be? Would I be a good mother? What did it even mean to be a good mother?

'A baby just needs a boob and a blanket,' Mara had told me. But she also emailed me a spreadsheet, passed down from expectant mother to expectant mother with rows of items that you needed post-birth. The items ranged from multiple pairs of black underwear and heavy sanitary pads (for the weeks of bleeding) to nappy bins that magically sealed away the smell of baby shit. You only had to wade into the shallow end of the internet to discover all the things you *should* own. The stuff that would build a wall to keep out the anxieties around forthcoming motherhood.

There were video monitors with night-vision-style technology which showed your sleeping baby in the dark, lit up in green like a heat-seeking missile; there were specific types of bottles with various teat sizes; and there were sterilisers, breast pumps, nipple shields, cribs and cots (which ranged from the standard, cheap IKEA model to a bassinet that could sense your baby waking and rock them back to sleep – which cost a cool $2000).

There were sleepsuits that bound your baby's arms by its side (to mimic the womb) and made your infant look like a pastel-coloured bat, wings drawn. There were pretty artisanal mobiles that hung above their bed and wall decals for a nursery that said things like *Sweet Dreams*. There were cocoon mattresses that were featherlight and could easily be scooted around the house so that your infant could sleep in the laundry or the kitchen while you continued to do chores.

Everything tacitly promised to smooth the terrifying journey ahead. It was the Mount Everest kit of motherhood. The difference being that on Mount Everest you were expected to pack light, on Mount Motherhood, you could never have enough – forever lugging a nappy bag and wipes and clean onesies and bibs and dummies and on and on the list went.

I planned to use hand-me-downs and second-hand stuff as much as possible, friends had given me an old pram and others had given me bags of used clothes, but there were still things that I would have to buy.

'You should have a baby shower,' Lucie said. 'Go on. You need all the baby shit. For all the baby shit that's coming.'

I screwed up my face, picturing saccharine games and pastel cupcakes and nappies smeared with melted chocolate bars and an all-female guest list.

She read my mind.

'It'll be low key, I can organise it.'

My fortieth birthday was coming up and I decided to make it a combined party so there would be less emphasis on the shower and more on the milestone of aging. Instead of birthday presents, people could buy something for the baby. But even if it was low key, there was the problem of hiring a venue and food and drinks and the cost. Perhaps my parents could host the party at their spacious house? But I wasn't sure which mother I would encounter when I asked: the generous, sociable mother or the tight-lipped, disapproving mother.

A month and a half before my fortieth birthday, on a cool June night, if you'd peered through the windows of my parents' house, you would have seen a gas fireplace glowing. In front of the fire, a pregnant woman was curled on the floor, letting the heat warm her back. The room was lit by floor lamps and bright green curved retro couches piled with large cushions. There were clean white tiles and a cream rug and bright, splashy art on the walls. On the couches, sat my family: my mum and my dad and my brother Tom. If you pressed your face to the cold windowpanes, it was elegant and inviting but inside sat almost forty years of tricky history. And burrowed inside my mother and me were our animal selves, coiled tight and ready to strike.

I dragged my heavy body to sitting and asked, as casually as possible, what my mum thought about having a party at their house.

'I'm not a fan of baby showers.' Mum's face was pinched.

There was part of me that knew I should leave the subject there. But I pressed on.

'It could be fun. Nothing saccharine. And you can invite some of your friends too, if you want.'

At this, her eyes narrowed. I'd made a terrible misstep.

'You're not to ask my friends for things. Like money for your musical.'

This was a sharp swerve sideways and I couldn't help taking the bait.

'It was a fundraising campaign, they were donating to a theatre production.'

'It was embarrassing.' Her face was dark. My body became rigid. The room felt like it had filled with dense, heavy weather. Tom edged into the kitchen to avoid what was to come.

'People think we can't provide for you,' my dad chipped in.

'You don't need to provide for me. It was a fundraising campaign for a theatre production. I wasn't forcing anyone to donate.'

'You're not to ask my friends for anything ever again.' Mum's words were bitter stones.

A swirling rage took hold of me, I stood up. 'I'm almost forty, I don't need to ask your permission.'

'Exactly you're an almost-forty-year-old who doesn't care about your parents at all,' she spat at me.

'All I do is care about what you think, I'm always trying to please you. And I find it hurtful that you don't want to celebrate me or the baby.'

'It's not hurtful.'

'I feel like it *is* hurtful.'

'You think you can put the words "I feel" in front of any sentence and say whatever you like.' She looked at me with triumph. Her intellect had won.

I felt the fury of a thousand childhood rebukes. The endless spun-out madness of being told I was asking for too much, that I was too much, that I should box up my feelings and my swelling body. I opened my mouth and screamed at her, 'YOU'RE A CRAZY, FUCKING BITCH!'

The words flew across the elegant furnishings and landed on my mother, who for once, eyebrows arched in disbelief, had nothing to say. I turned and marched out of the house, as much as a pregnant woman can march – like an octogenarian power walker with a giant marshmallow stuffed between her legs.

I sat in the driveway in the car, wheezing sobs. In the dark outside, I saw Tom lope down the front steps. He opened the car door and ducked his head in.

'Are you okay?'

'Yeah, no, yeah ... She's insane.'

He raised his eyebrows in agreement. 'I love you, Al.'

My sweet baby brother.

'Thanks. I love you, too.'

Tom shut the door and made his way back into the house for the aftermath.

I replayed the words. *You're an almost-forty-year-old who doesn't care about your parents at all.* This wasn't about a baby shower. It was about straying outside the lines of convention: becoming a single mother, asking for help. The message was clear: I was not to ask for things. To show need. Stoicism and self-sufficiency were the order of my family. I had ignored the rules. Of course, now that I was having a baby alone, I would have to ask for help, often.

As I drove back to my friend's house, the windscreen fogged and I couldn't stop crying. The roaring had vacated my body and now all that was left was sadness. Why was it so impossible for me and my mother to talk, to understand each other? Why couldn't I just let go of my lifetime of accumulated grievances towards her? I was an adult. Soon to be a mother. If we couldn't work it out, what kind of mother would I be to my son? Up ahead, the car lights bled together, smudged yellow and red, making it impossible to see.

Three of Us

On the weekend, I drove around the wide bend of Melbourne's Port Phillip Bay looking for somewhere to live. I felt myself disappear into the open sky and palm trees. I had lived in the north for most of my life in Melbourne and when I drove across the river, I missed the comfort of the cramped streets and Victorian cottages. Here wasn't home. But I needed to move south to be closer to my parents for help with the baby.

Instead of getting closer during my pregnancy, Mum and I were not speaking. Our relationship had always been fraught – each of us at either end of a delicate highwire constructed from politeness and surface talk that kept us at a distance. The taut line was now silent and slack between us but it was also thunderously loud. Our argument was the soundtrack to my waking days.

Was moving south a mistake? Maybe I should stay in the north, where most of my friends were instead.

There was the question of who I could rely on once I had a baby. Was it my friends who would be my ballast? Could I call them at the last minute if I ran out of nappies or needed a babysitter? Would they take on the burden and the love of what was to come? The friends with kids were overloaded with their own responsibilities. My single friends were living busy, social lives. Was it too much to ask them to be family? As a single woman, I had long been self-reliant. It was impossible to know who would step up; how I would have the courage to ask; what I could expect.

A week before my birthday, I got a text message from Mum.

Do you think we could find a way to get along? Now that the baby is coming.

It was like a blister bursting: pain and release. She had been the first to break. I knew that she was trying.

But I didn't want to reason with my parents alone – it would be two against one. I was afraid that things would end the way they had before. I decided to take control of the situation.

I went to see my GP who was a colleague of my mother's. In fact, Mum had recommended her. My GP had short grey hair and a gentle steadiness; she was thorough and considerate. She pulled a measuring tape over the hardened mound of my stomach – 'It's the most unreliable of the measurements but we do it anyway,' she said – as I explained the situation to her. She listened for a long time. 'I see,' she said finally. 'Your mother is worried about you.' She wasn't chastising me. She suggested some names of people I could call to help mediate.

I drove up to a terrace house south of the city one night after work and looked up at the shining lights in the windows. I closed my eyes and tried to count my breaths. My parents had agreed to meet with a therapist but this was not a conversation I wanted to have. Once we opened up what was between us, what terrible truths could come tumbling out? I forced myself to open the car door and heave my lumbering body out.

In a room that was all blush tones, my parents and I sat opposite a plump-faced therapist, her brows knitted with concern. I glanced at my parents' faces. My dad was definitely here under duress – a man who preferred few words. My mum's face was tender, uncertain. The room was cramped so that our bodies and the feelings they housed were too close for comfort.

'So what brings you here?' the therapist asked.

I took a breath and, in stops and starts, explained the situation as best as I could. My solo pregnancy. My parents' reticence. The explosive argument about the baby shower. The way I wanted my parents' support and encouragement.

'You have to understand,' Dad said. 'Our parents never encouraged us.'

'Never,' Mum agreed. 'When they visited us overseas when you were a baby, we had to do everything. To cook for them and show them around London.'

My parents shook their heads, smiling at the memory.

'We've tried to encourage you,' Mum said. 'We really have, I don't know if you see that.'

I was already stupidly crying.

'But you've been against the idea of me having a baby on my own. I feel like you're still disapproving,' I said.

'I'm just worried for you that it'll be hard.'

My mother paused and I saw that she was afraid. That her disapproval had been cloaking her fear. That her fear was an extension of her love for me.

'I'm just worried the baby will be sad that he doesn't have a father,' she said.

'There's three of us,' I said, drawing a circle between us with my hands. 'And that certainly hasn't protected us from sadness.'

My parents shifted uncomfortably.

'And why does it have to be sad? It should be joyous. It's your grandchild. It's a gift. We should be celebrating. That's why I wanted to have a party.'

'It's very hard to say no to you.' My mum sighed quietly. The words would normally have sparked anger but instead I saw a flicker of something that was to come: the insatiable hunger of a child; the ceaseless demands they make of their mother; my constant, unquenching need for love and attention. I was no longer angry. Something had softened and defused in that room.

I held my belly, where beneath my tightening skin a small creature swam. Was he oblivious to this sadness and anxiety? His amniotic fluid was probably spiked with the pain of his forebears. Poor bastard.

Screw you, I imagined him saying, as he kicked joyously against my body and the idiocy of his family. This child, I had a feeling, would be more resilient than any of us.

Afterwards, Mum hugged me tightly on the street. 'We love you and we'd like to take you out to dinner for your birthday,' she said.

I nodded, relieved.

Here was the mother I wanted to be, the loving and forgiving and generous mother.

A few weeks later, my friends and family gathered in a beer tavern that Lucie had managed to book for free. My brother Nick flew down from Sydney. My family paid for pizzas and ice-cream cake. Lucie made a long speech filled with embarrassing stories about our reckless university days and compliments that made me squirm.

Afterwards, I drove Lucie home. I was so tired, more swollen gourd than human. As we coasted down the High Street hill in Northcote, the glimmer of the city spread out below us, Lucie started yelling. The leftover ice-cream cake was melting in her lap. I stopped the car and we got out and sat in the gutter. She got a spoon and handed me one. And, like children, we ate the dripping sweetness straight out of the box.

The Lonely Woman

The front door to my new apartment building slammed loudly and I flinched. I'd finally found a place I liked on the south side of town: a small two-bedder on the ground floor with arched doorways, a courtyard and bright light that streamed in during the afternoon. Walking around the empty space at the rental inspection, I felt afraid but if I squinted I could make out my life there. And it was a short drive to my parents' house.

After years of sharing a house with other people, living alone was strange. I expected the door to open at any moment, for a housemate to arrive, to find me flustered and half-naked, rubbing body oil onto my distended belly. But no one was going to arrive – to enter from stage left through the door of my home and change the scene.

I had expected to feel relief at finally having a space to myself. Instead there was something else. Not fear but an itchy discomfort, a sense of not quite belonging. I wasn't lonely, that was the wrong word for it; I was jumpy, on edge.

Loneliness was a spectral character that had trailed me for years now. I wasn't lonely so much as afraid of the lonely persona that my single female life represented to the outside world. *She*, the character of loneliness, was single and pregnant; a sad

219

figure without a partner. In yoga class, she stared enviously at the glinting stones on the swollen ring fingers of the pregnant women. She was lonely but I had friends. She was lonely and her life was absent of meaning; but I had scenes and words to write for projects that filled me up.

She would be alone during her birth but I would not.

I hadn't figured out who would be with me during the birth though. I cycled through the options in my mind. My mother would either be too distressed by my pain or too detached – I imagined her swiping through Words With Friends on her phone in the corner of the labour ward. 'Yes, *Rioja*, one hundred and ten points!' she would say as I glared at her and moaned in pain.

'What? It's a Spanish wine!' she would reply.

I couldn't think of a friend who seemed like quite the right fit – the mothers were too busy with their children, the childfree like Lucie were too untested in matters of childbirth. But I wanted someone I felt comfortable with, someone who I knew. Sam suggested I hire a doula. A woman who was trained to support me before, during and, even possibly, post-birth.

I met Gab in a sparse room with wooden floorboards and clean walls at a space she'd started in Melbourne's west. It was a Meet the Doulas gathering. Each of the six doulas explained how they worked while the small circle of pregnant women listened.

Gab spoke in a calm, clear voice and made eye contact with each of us. 'First and foremost, as doulas, we're here to anticipate what your needs are in the birth space and in the motherhood space and fill the gaps of the mainstream maternity system,' she said. 'Women are expected to know what to do during birth,' she continued. 'No one prepares us though. We're all feeling out of depth when it comes to birth.'

Yes. Precisely, I thought, thinking of the vague terror that hovered around what lay ahead.

'As doulas, we're there to protect your space in pregnancy and protect your space in birth and make sure you're feeling safe and that the birth is on your terms.'

I'd been alone for so much of this process, I longed to be taken care of, to be protected.

Afterwards, when the circle had disbanded, I cornered Gab and introduced myself.

'I'm a solo mother by choice, my baby is donor conceived,' I told her. 'So I won't have anyone there with me during the birth.' Gab nodded but didn't blink. She didn't react with overt enthusiasm or dismay, simply took it in. It was the perfect response.

My own mother had sworn by an epidural and had one for all three of her children.

'What's your take on epidurals?' I asked.

'I think epidurals work beautifully for some people,' Gab said. 'It's a misnomer that doulas are only about homebirth and no interventions. What I believe in is having a mother who is supported and is birthing on her terms.'

I wanted someone who rated lower on the California-hippy-colour-chakras-and-patchouli-oil scale and higher on the pragmatism-and-supportive-lack-of-judgement-to-whatever-kind-of-birth-I-fucking-wanted scale. Gab was genuine. There was not a whiff of chakra-talk about her yet her demeanour felt almost spiritual in its clarity.

As we talked, I understood that Gab would be there for me no matter what, that she would support me during my pregnancy and my birth. I wanted desperately to work with her. Before I'd arrived, I barely knew what a doula was and now I needed her. She agreed that we could work together, and she said she would go to hypnobirthing class with me.

Hypnobirthing – or calm birthing – appealed to me. The stories I'd ingested from my mother about labour were all agony and horror and near death. But I'd heard a hypnobirthing expert talk about how hypnobirthing prepared women for a positive and empowering birth. Hypnobirthing, contrary to how it sounded, wasn't about being hypnotised during birth – it was about finding a state of relaxation during labour. It was about reducing fear and therefore tension and pain during contractions. The idea that you could master your fears around birth to have a positive, meditative experience seemed slightly whacky but not too whacky – which I guess is the scale that I live on.

I had emailed the hypnobirthing teacher to explain that I was a solo parent and asked if her class would be inclusive. She had assured me it would.

॰ᐇ॰

Gab and I filed into the semi-circle of hard plastic chairs. Around us were straight couples. The space was gallery white. We went around the room doing introductions. 'This is my doula, Gab,' I said to answer the question on all of the couples' open, nervous faces.

The hypnobirthing teacher was pale with thin lips and dark

red lipstick. She had a soft, pinched way of speaking. 'Okay, we're going to start with a video,' she said.

Onto the white wall a projection appeared: a floral graphic over pan flutes. We all sat silently watching as the video cut to a woman labouring in a bath. She was quiet as could be. A man sat by the side of the bath holding her hand. The baby flowed out of the woman without her making so much as a peep. I looked around the circle. Were people buying this bullshit? The scene faded away to an angelic pan flute finale.

'So how did you feel about that?' The teacher smiled encouragingly and looked around the circle. I could hear the men sighing with relief. 'That doesn't look bad at all,' one man said. The other men all nodded. The women looked sceptical.

I put my hand up. The teacher nodded at me. 'I'm just wondering about pain relief … epidurals?' I asked. The teacher's face twitched with disapproval. She reminded me of my high school history teacher when I'd asked why humans had decided to wear clothes. My history teacher had wrinkled her nose and said, *For decorum.*

The other women in the circle were eagerly waiting for an answer to my question. 'We'll get to interventions later,' the teacher said. 'First we're going to start with an exercise.' She held up a piece of paper with a tree drawn on it. 'I want you to write down all your fears about birth on the branches of this tree.'

When we had finished silently scribbling our endless fears, the teacher passed around a rubbish bin. 'Put your fears in the rubbish!' she said as though that was that.

She went on to explain that hypnobirthing was all about banishing fear. To not even say the word. Hypnobirthing replaced the words *contraction, pain, fear* with *wave, pressure, intensity*. Get rid of fear, the message was, and birth will be bliss. I wanted to believe it, I wanted to banish my fear, but during the tea break another expectant mother and I compared notes.

'It's like I have to become a Zen master in two months. And this shit takes people lifetimes,' I said.

The other mother nodded, my fear reflected in her eyes.

She looked at me curiously. 'It's great you're here with your doula.' I could tell she wanted to ask why my partner wasn't here. I was too tired to get into it, so I just smiled.

'It is great.'

Since becoming pregnant, I'd often encountered the questions and curiosity of others. Sure, single mothers had always existed but the consciousness and deliberateness of single women using donor sperm to take their reproductive future into their own hands was still relatively new.

According to the Victorian Assisted Reproductive Treatment Authority, single women in my state were the largest group to use donor sperm to conceive – ahead of same-sex couples. And in 2022, for the first time, the Australia and New Zealand Assisted Reproduction Database had taken into account family diversity and included single women and same-sex couples in their 2020 annual report. It found that 10.2 per cent of treatment cycles were done by single women (that included egg freezing and donor conception).

It was hard to pin down actual numbers of solo mothers globally because no one had done a count. But on the website of the world's largest sperm bank, Cryos, they touted the fact that more than 50 per cent of women who ordered sperm from them were single mothers-to-be. Based on doctors' reports, the explosion of news articles, fertility TikTok influencers, solo mum celebs and the growing numbers in solo mothers' groups online, I was part of a rising tide of women.

While solo motherhood was becoming more common, it still aroused curiosity. Most people's questions to me seemed to conceal another series of questions, a series of judgements. *Were you so desperate to be a mother that you chose to do it alone? Is it lonely? And are you scared? And most of all: how did you get here?*

How *did* I get here? Was it destiny or chaos, misfortune or luck that had led me past the prerequisite of coupledom to motherhood? The creation of a life was the ultimate experiment in causality. It felt random and miraculous. How did one of the million spermatozoa swim to the egg and bullseye? How had the fertilised egg survived through these uncertain months in the womb so that it could emerge as a squalling, suckling creature? How would something that started as a flicker unfold into a man elbowing his way through a packed train?

Among the growing number of the solo motherhood, we often laughed at the many questions and blunders we encountered. Before I was pregnant, a pharmacist had advised me loudly in the aisle of the chemist: 'You should get your husband's sperm tested before you buy pre-natal vitamins.' Another solo mum had been irked by family members who called the egg donor her child's 'real mother'. To add to that, there were the administrative relics, like the patient forms that required you to name a partner or a 'head of household', implying that a man was still in charge.

I knew the assumptions and questions were driven by plain curiosity, but I didn't always want to explain the story of my life to strangers. If I had a male partner, I wouldn't need to explain my pregnancy. Bound to a man, I'd be armoured and shielded by convention. It was clear that we didn't yet have the right words for our new families.

∙◦∙

After the tea break, the hypnobirthing teacher waxed lyrical about the warm and fuzzy feelings that birth induced.

'There'll be a lot of oxytocin in the birthing room,' she said. 'Just like the atmosphere in the bedroom when you're making love.'

My doula, Gab, and I tried not to catch each other's eye in case we started laughing.

'And your husband …'

The teacher looked at me and corrected herself.

'I mean, birth partner is there to bring you back to the breath.'

During lunch, Gab and I walked to a café.

'I should probably find a husband to shower me with love during labour.' I glanced at Gab, trying to make light of my anxiety.

'Don't worry,' Gab said, 'I'll be there to love you.' She looked me straight in the eye. 'You won't be alone.' Her words were perfect. She meant every one.

Gratitude

The obstetrician at the hospital was looking at my file when she saw something she didn't like. 'You're forty!' She shot me a disapproving look. 'You should have been getting scans every week, because of your age.'

At thirty-six weeks pregnant, at one of my final appointments, this was news to me. 'We need to book you in for a scan *now*, because of your age.' A zip of terror ran up my spine that quickly turned to fury as she continued tut-tutting over my file. I nodded at what she was saying, swallowing my annoyance.

I was, through luck at my baby's good health so far and my own hubris, disbelieving of the obstetrician's alarm. At each of my appointments and scans – the glucose test, the urine tests, the blood tests, the checks for the heartbeat, the measurements, the weigh-ins – my GP had assured me that the baby was going well. There had been some minor blips – a rash on my leg and stomach that could have been a build-up of bile salts but wasn't, a low ferritin reading which meant I needed to start eating meat, the ongoing pain in my pelvis, but all of it, I was assured, was nothing to worry about.

I was hoping to go into labour naturally – even if I went beyond my due date – so I'd come to the appointment armed with my kind student midwife, Rachael, also a solo mum by choice, and a number of questions.

'I was wondering what the risk is of going over forty weeks? The likelihood of stillbirth?'

'I don't know, google it.' The obstetrician waved the question away with her hand. I imagined googling the words *stillbirth* and *risk* and *forty weeks* and my terror unspooling along the dark threads of the internet.

'If you were my private patient, I wouldn't let you go over forty weeks. Because of your age.' I felt chastised, again, for being old.

The obstetrician asked who would be supporting me during my labour. I gestured at Rachael, and explained that my doula, would also be there. I told her that my son was donor conceived. At this the obstetrician became inspired.

'Do you know how hard it is?' she asked, then answered her own question. 'It's *very* hard.'

I wasn't sure if she was talking about labour or solo parenting. Rachael was murmuring in agreement. Out of politeness, I hoped.

'Do you know how many African women die in childbirth? Natural selection!' the obstetrician said triumphantly.

My brain was trying to scramble together a sentence of protest but I couldn't think, I was too shocked to assemble words. I'd arrived feeling tired but composed, eager for reassurance and updates on the imminence of my baby's entrance into the world. Now I could feel my eyes stinging but I didn't want to cry in front of this woman, to let her see any of myself. I wanted to stand up and roar like a sumo wrestler and hurl my giant belly at her, squashing her flat. Instead, Rachael and I politely murmured our thank-yous and exited into the packed waiting room filled with pregnant women and toddlers running in mad circles. We stood and looked at each other, shaking our heads. 'What was that?'

'Seriously. And did she really have to mention your age so many times?' asked Rachael, who conceived her two sons solo after forty. She hugged me tightly and hurried off to university.

I lined up at the reception desk and waited until it was my turn. I told the receptionist that I'd like to make a complaint about the obstetrician. The receptionist nodded with knowing sympathy as I gave her the obstetrician's name and then she directed me to the room where I could lodge a complaint. I looped the halls in a slow shuffle. I hated doctors, I thought to myself as I walked in circles. I hated their lawyer-like forecasting of worst-case scenarios, I hated their negative prognoses, I hated their scaremongering.

I realised on my third loop around the purple-carpeted halls that I was lost. I could barely walk more than ten steps without being in agony – my pelvic pain had grown worse these last few months – so I eventually gave up and went to wait for my scan. I was too tired to make a fuss.

In the ultrasound room, the man doing the scan had no lust for life – as though being sequestered in this dark space, running a machine over women's bellies all day had leached him of joy. He answered my questions in a clipped, disinterested tone. 'The baby looks fine. His head is engaged.' I marvelled at how something so miraculous – seeing a tiny being moving beneath a person's skin – could become so pedestrian to this sonographer.

In the lift, I watched my belly as the boy rippled across it, pushing down on my bladder and my belly button, which had popped out. I couldn't tell if it was his hand waving at me or his foot kicking against the limits of his confinement. He was engaged, somehow his head had slipped down into my pelvis without my noticing.

The baby was ready; poised to exit into the world and claim it as his own. But I felt less than ready in every way. My hospital bag was not packed. My apartment was still half empty; I had no bassinet yet. The baby clothes that had been handed down to me still needed to be sorted into different sizes and put away in drawers. I had three weeks to get everything ready.

That evening, I swayed down a pitch-black driveway and shut the door against the sharp cold of late winter and let myself be swaddled by the warmth and low lighting of a yoga studio. There was the waft of burning Palo Santo and chanting over the speakers. The teacher asked the circle of pregnant women, whose ripening bodies were propped up by numerous bolsters and blocks, to go around and describe how we were feeling.

'I am so consumed by my physical body, it's boring,' I said.

A woman next to me inhaled and exhaled slowly then beamed, 'Grateful. I'm grateful to be sitting here, in a position where I'm not in pain.'

I immediately regretted my own description. I wish I'd invoked gratitude. Instead, I felt constantly frustrated and sore and cranky. In bed, my pelvis ached and when I woke in the middle of the night, in order to turn over I had to get onto all fours to awkwardly move from one side of my body to the other. My stomach was covered with an itchy rash. Each day it was getting harder to walk the ten or so steps from the work carpark to my desk. Thankfully, my boss had agreed to let me park in the spots that were reserved for management so that I didn't have to traverse a number of blocks to reach my office.

At work, I was tired and irritable. When my colleague told me off for munching on toast at my desk because eating at our desks was against office policy, I snapped at him: 'Are you really telling me I have to walk all the way down to the kitchen to eat this?' Then I turned and shuffled angrily down the now epic flight of stairs to reach the kitchen.

Later at home, I watched the BBC's *Little Women* and felt weepy that I didn't have a Teddy Laurence to love me unequivocally. Someone handsome and true. I unpacked a standing lamp a friend had sent me and sat perched on a fit ball trying to assemble it, but the top part evaded me, I couldn't get it to fit together.

I lay on the couch, one hand on an icepack for my tingling fingers that were deadened with the numbness of carpal tunnel caused by pregnancy. I was ready for bed by 7 pm. Ready for the coming rain. Ready for relief. Ready for this baby to arrive so I could walk again.

I ate a cob of corn slathered in butter and watched pieces fall onto the floor and didn't bother to pick them up. I imagined all the other women, sitting alone in their apartments, pregnant. Were they worrying about money? Did they often do sums in their head, counting out the weeks of minimum-wage paid parental leave and trying to figure out how they'd stretch their savings beyond that for maternity leave? Did they worry about how they'd have to return to work after three months because they were the sole earner? Did they think about who and when someone would next kiss them on the neck? Were they afraid too?

For one gulping ache, I longed for someone to cook me dinner, stroke my hair and place their hand on my belly to feel *our* baby kicking. Romance and the possibility of it seemed to have floated off into the ether.

My ringing phone interrupted my thoughts: Sam's grinning face appeared on my screen. She had recently broken up with a woman she'd been dating.

'Hey … How are you feeling?' I answered.

'It sounds terrible, but I feel kind of relieved,' she said.

I heard her son Loki in the background – now a toddler.

'Time to sleep, Lokes, come on.' There was a whine of protest and then a door shutting.

Sam scrabbled the phone back to her ear.

'Bedtimes are tricky at the moment … what was I saying?'

She caught me up on her life, the break-up, the revelation she'd recently had.

'I had this moment where I realised I'm one of the first generations of women who can be financially stable on their own, have a child on their own. That I'm not required to partner up for financial or any other sort of security. And like, what an absolute privilege and joy.'

I loved Sam's optimism and the way she always tilted my perspective so that I was viewing an expanse of history rather than a sliver of my lonely evening. She continued on.

'So many women in history would never even imagine that this story is possible. And if we could go back and tell them, that this is possible, imagine the joy they would feel.'

As she spoke the words, I saw centuries of women in crinolines and tight corsets and binding footwear watching me from the walls of my apartment. They were wide-eyed, gleeful. I imagined their laughter in a tinkling chorus of wonder at this new world.

I saw them all, and realised that I had something that they did not. I was free.

Power of Two

Friday, 5 pm

In the bathroom at work, I noticed some splotches of red on my underwear. I was exactly thirty-seven weeks pregnant; it was my last day of work. I felt lousy. Exhausted. 'I hope it's not labour,' I joked to my colleague whose eyebrows shot up in fear.

The owner of the company who was visiting from Sydney overheard and swaggered over to give me some advice. 'During labour, what you need is for your husband to shake some Tic Tacs at you. And play some music with no lyrics. Get your husband to distract you from the pain.'

'I'll have to find a husband.' I smiled.

'Oh, I'm sorry,' he replied, while not sounding at all sorry.

I managed to just make it through to the end of the day. Then I limped down the stairs clutching a big white giftbox filled with miniature white clothes and drove away.

I got home and texted a photo of my bloodied underwear to my midwife, Rachael. She was unfussed: *Call the hospital, probably just the show which is nothing to worry about and a sign you're getting close*, she wrote. The show was the razzle-dazzle performance of the mucus plug coming away from the uterus. I called the hospital.

While I was on hold, I wandered into the nursery which had a double bed in it instead of a cot and only half a change table, still missing a cushioning mat for the top. As I paced slowly back to my bedroom, I looked at the space where the bassinet should sit next to my bed. It still hadn't been dropped off. First babies were always overdue. Surely, I still had time. I hadn't even done the hospital tour yet. A midwife finally answered. I filled her in. Her voice was as comforting as warm milk. 'Just stay home and wait. You can always call us if you're worried. You're not in labour yet.'

In those strange early hours between midnight and daylight I woke up to soft insistent spasms. An earworm played in my head, an old Indigo Girls song, 'Power of Two'. The song soothed me, everything would be okay, my baby and I would be fine. I turned on the light and timed the spasms. I couldn't remember how many minutes apart things were supposed to be. I called the hospital again. Another kind woman answered. The kind woman recommended painkillers and sleep.

Saturday, 11 am
The spasms had returned but I was strangely calm. I sway-walked around my apartment. Lucie dropped off food and brand-new leopard-print pyjama pants. My mum came by, bringing things I might need for hospital. She helped me pack my hospital bag, just in case.

'I hate to leave you when you might be in labour, but I have to go to the ballet this afternoon and then we're driving down to the coast to play golf,' she said. I shook my head, amused at my mother's roster of activities. I wasn't worried. I'd heard about early labour lasting for days.

'Why don't you call Tom?'

'I'm fine, really.' And I was. But after the door closed and I was on my own, I changed my mind. I called my brother Tom, and he agreed to come over. He was relieved to have an excuse not to go to his restaurant shift. He'd worked till 4 am and was wiped from the night before. We ordered Thai food. I propped my laptop on my bed and ate pad thai on all fours as I watched *Kath and Kim*. Occasionally a spasm would roll through my body and I'd stop chewing and try to breathe noisily through my mouth.

Saturday, 10.30 pm

I woke to a pop – a gush rushing out of me. I stood up, and water was flowing down my legs. The waves were really here now. I went into the spare room. Tom was lying in bed, asleep with all the lights on, his mouth open. I watched him for a second in my would-be nursery. The nursery that didn't even have a change table set up yet because I still had three weeks to set it up. 'Tom,' I said, suddenly feeling the urgency of what was happening. 'Tom, WAKE UP.' Tom's eyes jolted open. He got up and wandered around my apartment in a daze as I yelled instructions: 'Pillow! Hospital bag! Heat pack!' I stuffed a towel between my legs and clutched a hot water bottle to my middle.

'Go. Pull the car up out the front,' I said. I pulled a coat and scarf over my nightie and put on some woollen socks and pink high-top sneakers, looking truly mad. I waddled out of the apartment, towel wedged between my legs while I listened to a hypnobirthing meditation through my headphones (*Three, two, one, relax, relax, relax,* said an English woman's voice).

Tom's car was idling in the apartment block's one lane driveway. I was moving slowly. Everything had a distant, fuzzy quality – the headlights torched the silent plants and the stillness of the driveway.

I was trying to get into the car but I had to stop when a searing force rolled through my body. Just at that precise moment, as I was clutching the stars, the earth, the trees (or was it just the roof of the car?), another car pulled into the driveway in front of us and blocked our way. My neighbour, whom I couldn't make out through the dark, saw my doubled-over body, and quickly reversed out. Through the spasms, I inched my way into the passenger seat. The neighbour's car circled the block and drove in and out, in and out, in and out of the driveway. *Go away*, I thought. *Leave me alone.*

Saturday, 11 pm

The drive was interminable. I watched the lamplights blur as we passed by the lake just south of the city. Where were we? I felt disoriented. Was this a different city? We finally arrived at the hospital. My brother dropped me off while he went to park. I limped out into the neon-lit emergency driveway and through the sliding doors. A security guy looked up from an empty desk with disinterest. 'You've gone through the wrong door,' he said, barely looking up as he pointed to a different entrance. I clutched the sofa as a ballast and internally cursed his indifference as the force rolled through me again.

I exited and found myself in the right waiting room. It was blessedly empty. A woman whisked me into a room to examine me. I felt nauseous and someone quickly shoved a cardboard bowl under my mouth. Up poured a stream of acidic pad thai into the bowl. My brother reappeared.

'Can you rub my back?' I asked him. I leant over, elbows on the bed, while Tom kneaded my back.

'This is my brother,' I told the nurse.

'Ah … You'll always remember this,' she said to him.

She measured my contractions.

'You're labouring. Three minutes apart. If there's anyone you want here, you should call them now.'

They wheeled me up to the birthing suite in a wheelchair, at some point my brother peeled away into the darkness of the corridor. He would sit in that room until 4 am, patiently waiting, eventually going home after realising some hours later that the birth was not about to happen at any second.

My doula, Gab, arrived. Somehow she had appeared within minutes of my texting her. She took my hand. 'You can do this.' Immediately affirming. Then Rachael, the student midwife, was there. I reached for her hand too. I couldn't focus on the two women but I could feel them there, beside me.

Sunday, 12 am

I was lying in a bath. In the corner sat the hospital midwife. Her hands were folded on her stomach. The three women were circled around me. When the force rolled through me, Rachael and Gab incanted: 'You can do it, you're doing a great job, that's it!'

Over and over, words of encouragement and affirmation.

My teeth clamped down on the plastic bit of the gas machine and I inhaled. 'Suck in hard,' said the midwife. 'You want to hear the machine rattle.' The machine made a death rattle as I sucked.

I started to feel the gas loosen me. A dizzy lightness. Not so much relief, but distraction.

But still there were thoughts. Could I do this? Would I be a good mother? What if I wasn't enough? But then, like an LSD trip, the gas started to unravel everything into a tipsy, slow-motion revelation.

I need to be free of thought, I realised, big-eyed, sucking on the gas greedily. *I need to be free of thought*, the revelation widened, *not just now but ALWAYS! Because there's only LIFE, nothing else matters.* An invisible choir of angels started to sing as the answer to everything floated into me. I sucked more gas, seeking out the truth, like a stoned frat boy stumbling on the meaning of existence.

The choir crescendoed and I was rolling thunder, rolling agony. I was high and blank and my thoughts were gone. Then I was throwing up into another small cardboard bowl. Pieces of noodle sprayed out and hit the surface of the bathwater, but I didn't give a fuck. I was the way, the truth and the life.

The force rolled in and I whimpered but I wasn't afraid. 'What's happening?' I asked the midwife. She put the Doppler into the bath to measure the baby's heartbeat. She placed it on my stomach. Whoosh. Whomp. Galumph. Whoosh. Whomp. Galumph. 'Everything's fine, you're fine, the baby's fine,' she said.

Rachael showered my head. Gab fed me cold sips of water from a glass. The tap was turned on, more hot water was added to the bath. The sound of gushing water scraped up my back like sandpaper. My vision had tunnelled to a point. I was animal, nothing else.

Sunday, 7 am

The midwife said I needed to go to the bed to be examined. I didn't know how I would get from the bath to the bed – it was an impossible distance. At least three metres. A hot towel was wrapped around me, giving me comfort as I heaved myself across the room. The midwife examined me. I glanced up at Gab occasionally and locked eyes.

'You're doing so well. You're going to meet your baby soon,' she said.

Her words jolted through me. What if I wasn't ready to meet the baby?

'I need you to tell me I'm going to be a good mother,' I said.

Rachael and Gab laughed but it was a kind laugh.

'You're going to be a wonderful mother,' Gab said.

'You absolutely will be,' said Rachael. 'I have no doubt.'

'It's time to push,' the midwife informed me. I was fully dilated. It was too late for pain relief, too late for an epidural and they were confiscating my beloved gas. The midwife was instructing me. 'Hold your breath and push down like you're constipated.' I tried but each time I pushed, a fear-tipped flame ran through my lower back, my body tensed up, certain the pushing was going to unleash a tidal wave of agony.

I was ordered into different positions. I hung from a bar, squatting on the ground, hands held above my head. Then I was on all fours. Now I was lying sideways, someone holding my leg up. The pushing felt impossible. Arduous. Long. 'Just one more. Just one more. Just one more,' the room was chanting at me. But it'd been two hours of pushing and I still hadn't met my baby yet.

It was impossible. The baby wasn't going to come out. Perhaps he knew that I doubted that I would be a good mother. He knew and he was refusing to move from womb to earth.

Sunday, 9 am

All the lights snapped on. An obstetrician was at the foot of the bed. The room was suddenly a-hum with nurses and movement, everything beat faster. The obstetrician was perfectly made up: heavy false lashes, layers of cream and contoured cheekbones. Maybe she felt she needed to counter the sweaty and ugly grunting form of womanhood in front of her by appearing perfect. 'I need to do an examination.' Her gloves were on.

A machine was wrapped around me to track the heart rate. The baby's heartbeat had been clear and steady all this time. But now, all the calm had been sucked from the room and the baby's heart rate had dropped. 'We need to get the baby out,' the obstetrician said.

Gab looked at me, intently, willing me to push the baby out.

'Let's try pushing again, one more time,' I said.

'Do you need anything?' a nurse asked me kindly.

'A gin and tonic,' I said, trying to smile.

'There she is,' said Gab, because it was the first joke I'd made in nine hours.

I pushed and everyone was yelling: 'That's it! You're doing it! He's coming. He's just there! I can see his hair! Just one more!' But when I stopped pushing, the baby seemed to get swallowed back up again and I was getting tired of *just one more* push.

'Everything's okay,' Gab said. 'You're okay, the baby's okay. Keep focusing on your breathing.'

'Everything is NOT OKAY,' the doctor snapped. 'We need to get this baby out NOW.'

It didn't matter whether I believed that I was going to be a good mother or not, this baby was coming out. He had no time for my doubts.

'The baby is in the right position. I'm going to put a vacuum cup on his head,' the doctor said.

I heard her saying words, 'Now. Vacuum. Sting.' Then: 'PUSH!'

I pushed. A radical stinging zipped through me as the baby was sucked outwards.

'Breathe. Breathe. Small push, like a cough. Breathe,' she was saying. The room was ringing with a high pitch of wonder, a gasp. They had all seen his head.

It seemed like years. I'd thought he would just slip out in one go. But now, again: 'PUSH!'

'You can reach down and pull him out,' the doctor said.

I pulled up a small, slippery creature from between my legs.

He was on my chest. Someone was rubbing the white stickiness off his body with a towel.

'Oh God, oh God, oh God,' I heard myself say.

I felt my body fill up with all of it – the labour, the rolling sensation, the nausea, the sheer grunting force of pushing. All of it ran down my neck and along my back and out of me. I could cry. 'That's right, let it all out,' a voice said. But I wasn't crying. I was staring at the little thing on my chest.

A tiny boy, a person. The two of us were bloody. He shook and shuddered. His eyes were black slits, his hair dark tufts. His mouth opened and closed like a fish hooked from the sea. Love was too small a word. He was mine. He was mine. He was mine.

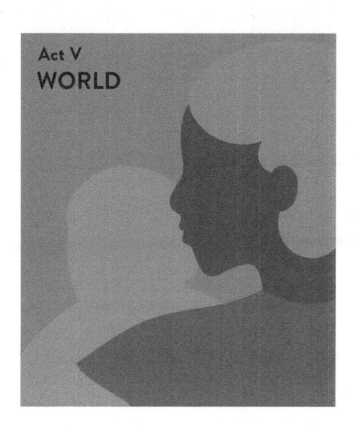

Act V

WORLD

Fourth Trimester

I was lying with the baby latched to my breast. His body was red and scrunched and speckled with placenta, his head cone-shaped from being sucked out by the vacuum. He was already asleep: half an hour of being alive was exhausting. Gab sat by the bed. We had retold the story of the birth already and now we were companionably silent, when a nurse popped her head around the door. 'Your parents are here.'

'Here, now?' I was confused about where they had materialised from. It was barely 9 am on a Sunday morning.

'Hi, darling,' Mum and Dad chorused as they walked into the room. 'Are you okay?'

There was a frazzle around them, but they stood at a shy distance, afraid to get too close. I had blood smeared on my chest and my face. I was naked under the sheets and the baby was still attached to my breast.

'How did you get here?' I asked.

'Tom called us last night. So we got up early and drove back from the coast,' Mum said.

'Without playing any golf?' I teased but a tenderness for my parents filled me up.

I briefly relayed the highlights of the labour reel: bath, gas, no time for an epidural, vacuum and now this creature. They exclaimed – 'amazing, incredible!' – and shook their heads, part disbelief, part wonder.

'Do you want to see him?' I asked. My dad stayed sitting by the window. But my mum inched over to the bed and cooed. 'Ohhh, look at him.' She put a tentative hand out to touch his head, not wanting to disrupt the closeness of his skin to my skin. Then she retreated back to sit by the wall. It was not the union of souls I'd been hoping for but nothing could undo my post-birth high.

'We were thinking,' Mum said, 'that maybe you should come stay with us for a while?'

'You'll need some help.' Dad looked gravely at me.

I was too blurry to absorb what they were saying.

'We'll let you … We'll go and come back tomorrow.' Mum stood up.

They left and I stared at this boy who had been cleaved from my body. Gab interrupted my reverie. 'Go stay with them. Take the help.' She looked at me, her face filled with a truth that I didn't yet understand.

I woke in the hospital the day after the birth to the buzz of women's voices down the hall – the caffeinated midwives going to and fro. I stayed cocooned in my room, with my son lying in a transparent plastic crib next to me. In the rooms around me, although I never once saw them, I imagined the other women, shellshocked, bleeding, beside their strange newborns. We had been wrenched in two, mothers and children, foreigners in a new land. I barely knew where I was, who I was, but I knew the midwives were out there, protecting us.

On the second day I named him. Quinn. Meaning: wise, intelligent. From the Gaelic: 'descendant of Conn'. Con was the name of my Greek grandfather. Middle name: Wilson, my mother's maiden name. Quinn Wilson Collier. When my parents visited, they proudly recounted telling their friends their grandson's name and explaining its origins.

Night two. A long night's journey into more night. I think the nurses had taken pity on me as a single mother, because even though it was a public hospital they had given me my own room and let me stay a second night.

The grey light through the hospital window, the hum of generators, the midwives with different bright faces and Irish lilts. The tray lady who always thwacked down my dinner. Quinn sleeping on my breast. Quinn yowling – his little neck straining and reaching for an impossibility. All sensation seemed painful to him. The world too scratchy and bright and loud. His distress was unbearable.

'Now, tuck his body under your arm like a football,' the midwife said.

Quinn was squirming, as I tried to cradle his body, his wobbly head, and place it under my arm. My breast was a giant pudding, naked and pendulous. Quinn opened and closed his mouth trying to get at it.

'Now nose to nipple, nose to nipple. You want him to open his mouth wider,' she said.

The pose felt ridiculous, especially since I hadn't held a football for three hundred years. 'Maybe this is too ambitious,' I said.

'It's good to be ambitious.' The midwife was not having my doubt.

You have no idea, I thought. My life had been one long thread of ambition that had led me here, to thinking I could do *this*. Quinn clamped down on my breast and sucked. His mouth was not wide enough, a shooting pain tore through my chest.

'Let's try it again,' the midwife said.

Later, Tom slunk into the ward even though it was past visiting hours.

'I just walked in,' he said. 'No one even looked at me.'

I handed Quinn to Tom, and watched the two of them from the bed. Tom stared down at his nephew, who barely stretched from his hand to his elbow.

'He's just so … He's just so … He's just so …' Tom was shaking his head in wonder. 'Cute.' But I could see that the word was not enough. There were no words for this.

A shy doctor knocked on the open door. She was here to explain a series of things about *baby*. The doctor directed her entire monologue – 'baby this, baby that' – at my brother. Tom and I exchanged a brief glance, the faintest of sibling smiles that implied a shared mocking language. But both of us were too embarrassed to interrupt her and explain that he was not the father.

Each minute, I had so many questions for the midwives. Blood in his urine? Normal. Cluster feeding for five hours? Normal. Pinched, dagger-sliced nipples? Normal. Tests. Leaflets. Beeping. Code blue. Code green.

On the baby's chest was a pink blemish. 'What's that?' I asked the midwife in alarm. 'That's his nipple,' she said. Totally normal.

I woke to find Quinn shaking in tiny tremors. Not normal. I pressed the help button. The midwives rolled his plastic crib down the pink hallway to the newborn intensive care unit to check his blood sugar. I walked alongside in my slipper socks with rabbit ears. In the intensive care unit, through a doorway I saw a woman, her face melting towards the floor with sadness. This was not a good place. I wanted to leave, to swallow my small boy back into my body where he was safe.

We entered a small bright room. The doctor quizzed me on what medications I was taking. 'Hm, possibly withdrawals,' he said. *Please, please let him be okay.* He pricked Quinn's heel for blood. Quinn screamed and screamed – the sound ripped through my body. I wasn't allowed to pick him up until they had finished so I patted him but it wasn't enough – my arms felt useless as they rolled him back along the hallway. 'You'll need to stay another night,' the doctor told me. 'Until his blood sugar is back to normal. Then you can go home.'

Home. Where was that? The thought of leaving the midwives' orbit was terrifying. Should I stay at my parents' house?

Later, the tremors had stopped but Quinn wouldn't sleep. Was it daytime? Night-time? What did it matter? My eyeballs felt flayed. I pressed the help button, again. Another midwife appeared, a rotating cast of warm, bustling women I couldn't keep track of.

She looked at my wild expression.

'Do you want me to take him for an hour?' she asked.

'What will you do with him?'

'They sleep fine with us.' She shrugged.

She checked the name on his wrist tag. 'Babies have been mixed up in the past,' she said cheerily, then rolled him away.

I closed my eyes. I was being dragged down by a deep tidal drift. I tried to get out of the bed but I was pinned. Quinn was out there, somewhere, I needed to find him. There was a bloodcurdling scream caught in my throat. I dragged myself into the hospital corridor but I was back in the bed again. Must. Get. Out. Dragged myself out. Looped back. Pinned to the bed again.

Finally, I made it out, bursting into the brightly lit corridor. All the women – the mothers and the midwives – were gathered in a pastel huddle, whispering. No one wanted to tell me the truth. Something terrible had happened to a baby. My baby. I was a dead woman walking towards them about to find out. But now I was parachuting through rainforest. I could see the gnarled whorl of the tree trunks. My feet landed with a thud outside a hut. Inside was a family who would give me their baby because I had lost mine. My grief would become their grief and it would never end.

I woke up to the rattle of the cot being wheeled back in. Quinn was asleep, untroubled.

I tried to explain the hallucinogenic dreams to the midwife. She nodded.

'Sleep deprivation nightmares. I *do not* miss those.'

I fell asleep and woke sweating. Where was he? Just here. Beside me. Still beside me. I reached my arm out and placed it on his ribs: small chest rising, small chest falling.

My parents came to visit again. They both cradled Quinn, wrapped snug in his blanket. We took photos. My dad was beaming.

'So do you want to come stay with us?' my dad asked again.

'Sure, that'd be good.' I darted my eyes away, embarrassed that I needed this gift.

It was decided, I would sublet my apartment and stay with my parents for a while – that way I could have their help and afford to extend my maternity leave.

The next day, my dad came to pick us up and paced back and forth as we waited for an hour for another doctor to give us the all-clear. Finally, they told us that Quinn's blood sugar levels were normal. We had permission to leave. In the lift, my dad held Quinn greedily in his arms as we descended to the carpark.

We were all thumbs trying to strap Quinn into the car; his body looked so small in the seat. It was like strapping Thumbelina into a turbojet. I sat beside him and stared out the window and watched as people streamed over the sunlit pedestrian crossing next to the hospital. What did they do to it, this world that I once knew? I felt like an amnesiac trying to piece back together my memory of life before.

At Mum and Dad's house, they held Quinn while I quickly showered and ate. They brought me breakfast and lunch on a tray, cups of tea and glasses of water, as I sat and Quinn fed and fed and fed. I was a human drink. Mum and Dad were both filled with purpose and pleasure.

The first morning, I came out of the bathroom and my parents were standing over his bassinet, staring down at him, murmuring, their faces soft. I couldn't hear or make out what they were saying, it was that nonsense language that adults dissolve into around babies. They were rapturous. Their happiness coursed through me.

I stood in the doorway, and wanted to freeze this tableau for as long as possible. To deliver the picture to my past self and say, *Here, look.*

The next day, the maternal child health nurse came to visit. She was a stout woman with a permanent frown. She was looking at my file, confused. 'How did you procure this child?' she asked. *Procure?* As though my son was a live parrot I'd smuggled through customs.

'At Melbourne IVF?' I looked at her to see if I'd answered correctly.

She had a pursed look of disapproval. Quinn kicked his legs on the change table, eyes beginning to take in the world. As we were talking, I stepped away from the change table and the nurse lunged towards Quinn, arms outstretched towards him.

'See how I stepped over!' she said. 'Because babies roll.' I was in trouble. Quinn lay inert, blinking, months away from rolling.

Before she left, the midwife turned to me and said, 'You should only plan to do one thing a day. That's enough.' One thing. Did that include feeding and changing the baby on a permanent loop? I assumed the one thing she meant was something other than the constant keeping-him-alive domestic minutiae. One thing for myself. But I couldn't imagine how that would be possible.

It wasn't just the million things that always needed doing, there were a million new terms to learn: breast refusal, nipple confusion, cluster feeding, milk bleb, fourth trimester, the three S's (sleep, swaddle, shushing), mastitis, colic, womb sounds, fontanelle, meconium, colostrum, sticky eye.

Perhaps my one thing was writing in my journal by the light of my phone torch, which was facedown on the page so as not to wake the baby. I needed to write everything down because my brain was filled with static. The newness of it all felt like a revelation that I must pin to the page. I wrote to the sound of

Quinn's breath whistling like a thin reed through his nose and to waves crashing through the white noise player.

Perhaps my one thing was being able to go downstairs into the living room at night, after he was in bed, and stretch my body out on the floor. But I was in a constant state of vigilance. What if he stopped breathing? Or rolled off my bed where he fell asleep? What if a possum had crashed through the ceiling and crushed him alive? Weird calamities played out in a constant stream behind my eyes. I listened through the baby monitor to the sound of him breathing and remembered my mother telling me about how she used to strain to listen to me too through the monitor. She waited, her own breath held, for the sound of my breath, in and out.

Quinn woke at 2 am and yowled. He wouldn't settle. I walked back and forth in the twilight of the bathroom blasting the fan for white noise so that it felt like we were in an engine, about to take off. I walked in figure eights over the tiles, round and round in the shape of eternity. As one hour became two, I saw myself open the window, hold out his screaming body and drop him two storeys to the ground. The image flooded me with cold, violent horror. God, I needed sleep.

Finally, he settled back, eyelids fluttering, half open, lips pursed. He breathed in short bursts and grunts and little murmurs. I stared at him. How were we ever going to leave Mum and Dad's? How would I do the million and one things that it took to get through each day? I messaged Mara a stream-of-consciousness series of questions about swaddles and pumping milk and dummies. She was, typically, awake in the middle of the night with her daughter. *You sound like a mum who hasn't had much sleep,* she wrote. *Don't worry, it's intense right now, but it gets easier.* She was always at the end of the line, giving me much-needed advice that I valued over that of coupled mothers. She understood the unique madness of choosing this path, of what it took; we were alone together.

Each day, I walked back and forth across the patio in the backyard, dazed as he cried unceasingly. 'Babies cry an average of two to three hours a day in the first twelve weeks,' Mum told me. Jiggle, jiggle, jiggle, rock, rock, rock. *You only have to get through today,* I said to myself. And when that was too much: *You only have to get through this hour.* And then: *You only have to get through this minute, this second, this nanosecond.*

My friends visited and brought food and gifts. 'You did this, this was all you,' Lucie said as she held him to her chest – he was blanket-wrapped, a sleeping burrito. She was grinning. We both stared at his body, which was so small it stretched from my neck to my belly button. Barely fifty-four centimetres long.

'You must be loving having Quinn here,' Lucie said to my mum who emerged from the kitchen with cups of tea.

'Oh yes. If he moves home, we'll run down the driveway yelling, "Don't go! Please, come back!"' Mum was only half-joking but we all laughed. I felt a greedy swell of pride and relief. Now that Quinn was here, my parents were lovestruck.

All day, Quinn fed ferociously. His small quivering mouth sucked and sucked at my nipple. I tried to soften my body, exhale, while he drank, not wanting to feed him my worry. Sometimes as he fed he looked at me out of the side of his eye, sleepily keeping a bead on events. He slept with his fingers splayed across his eyes as though he was shielding himself from the paparazzi. He had a dark ring of hair at the base of his skull that made him look like a balding, 55-year-old accountant.

Each night, my dad said to the speaker, 'Hey Google, play "Mighty Quinn".' And he stood swaying with Quinn in his arms, bobbing up and down. My son wide-eyed, reed-thin arms flung around his grandpa's neck, head lolled over his shoulder, as Dad bopped up and down and gruffly serenaded the mighty Quinn. Or Dad played Van Morrison's 'Days Like This' and, oh my heart, who knew there'd be days like this watching my father with my son?

September became October, that in-between month. A bright spring headachy tired. Days and nights of feeding. His trembling lip, his thrashing arms signalling that he was about to wail at 3 am. I lifted him out of bed, his small ribs fitted in my hands so that the tips of my fingers touched. I propped myself up, turned the light on, attached him to my breast and read three pages of a novel that I'd never finish.

My brother Tom and I took turns sitting on the couch holding him in our laps and watched the weather of emotions ripple across his sleeping face. *Quinn TV*, we called it. In the mornings, I took Quinn into my parents' room and he laid between them on the bed, kicking his growing limbs as they talked to him in wonder-soft voices.

My brother Nick flew down from Sydney and stayed with us for a week. He went to my apartment and installed a washing machine he'd bought for me, sawing off pipes so it would fit and constructing my furniture that was still in boxes and pieces.

The days were indistinguishable other than the way the light fell through the window, by the sun warming us as it tracked closer to our patch of earth. In December, as I breastfed in the living room at dusk, my mum sat quietly on the bright green couch opposite me. 'He's perfect. You're doing all the right things.' I smiled at her, grateful.

I looked at him; my son. Awe expanded my lungs, my body leavened and grew to take him in. I was greedy for the beauty of him, the baby of him. Give me this psychedelic rush of togetherness any hour, any day: his fist curled around my finger, his mouth widening into a tiny yawn, the weight of his lolling head on my chest.

For a few minutes, I was able to forget that soon I'd be home, doing this alone. I had no idea how I could, how I would.

'I love you so much,' I whispered to his sleeping, flickering face. I would continue to say those words. *I love you*, beyond measure.

Just a Mother

I sat on the cold basement floor crying. Quinn was nine weeks old. It was the first day of parents' group. I was eager to meet other parents – to find people to share the madness of this time with. But I'd spent the last thirty minutes trying to put together the pram. The unyielding metal legs of the pram were like crocodile jaws, clamped shut. I kicked them and threw the pram and myself to the floor, swearing and crying. If I couldn't do this one thing, how was I going to do anything on my own? I gave up and went upstairs and asked my dad for help.

After these past months at my parents' house, I now heard an edge in my mother's voice when she asked if I wanted dinner. The shine of newborn excitement had worn off. Or perhaps I was turning into my teenage self, projecting my resentment at having reverted to childlike helplessness around my parents.

I needed to return to adulthood, to remember who I was. I needed to learn how to be a mother on my own. But what if I couldn't do it? What if I couldn't survive without meals being made for me and breaks when my son was being held by others? Or was it that the longer I stayed, the less capable I was becoming?

After Dad had assembled the pram, I made my way to the parents' group at the local day care centre. The women sat in a circle, each with a barnacle attached. Behind us, through the windows, toddlers swarmed through the sunshine, yelling and playing at the adjoining kindergarten but we were too laser-focused on our barnacles to notice.

One woman was draped in a muslin wrap for modesty as she breastfed, another was jiggling her pram with a manic expression that was akin to a bank robber mid-heist. Chloe, who had brown-grey curls frizzing around her face, was on the floor changing her baby's nappy. I immediately liked her because of the dry way she described her daughter Greta as a 'mini Mussolini'. Everyone was wide-eyed, trying to smile brightly through the shock of our arrival at motherhood.

The nurse sat at the front of the room and took us in with a Hollywood-wattage beam. She was in her element – the doyenne, the knowledge keeper for this shambling group of women. She enunciated her words as though each fact she was imparting was a revelation: 'Babies sleep in forty-five-minute cycles!', 'Hiccups are a sign of tiredness!', 'You're not going to believe it but the best thing for cradle cap is … *(hold for tension)* … OLIVE OIL!'

The nurse asked us to pair up and play an icebreaker. We were to explain to the stranger sitting next to us the origin story of our baby's name. I paired up with a woman who had brought her husband – the only man in the room. The pair told a well-worn story, gushing about the negotiations that went into deciding on a name together. I explained to them the origin of Quinn's name. My speech, unlike theirs, was prefaced with *I* not *we*. Were the husband and wife wondering why no one else was consulted about my son's name?

I hadn't told the group that my son was donor conceived. It wasn't exactly that I was avoiding telling them. Or was I? I was relieved that all the talk here was taken up with obsessive worry about tummy time and sleep cycles and dribble rash. In this room, I didn't need to qualify; I belonged. I was just another mother.

'I'm not *just* a mother,' Chloe said to the group as we talked about our new, shattered identities. But even if I wasn't *just* a mother, I was always a mother. If your child was with someone else, and you were at work, you were a mother. If your child was an adult, you were a mother. If your child had passed away or you'd miscarried, you were a mother. The mother-ness of you was always and everywhere.

'Now, let's talk about sex,' the nurse said. The circle of women were silent but riveted. 'You want to get your partner to aim *high*.'

I said nothing.

'I haven't been able to brave it yet.' Chloe giggled.

Nobody else said a word.

In the break, as we drank tea and hoovered down shortbread creams, ravenous from breastfeeding, a woman with silky brown hair turned to me. 'So, are you and your partner staying with your parents?'

I shook my head. 'I don't have a partner. Quinn is a donor baby.'

'Oh, that's great. Good on you,' she said her voice rising to a nervous pitch.

I was exposed and relieved. My secret was out.

Later, Chloe and I ambled home in the sun pushing our prams.

'Do you have a partner?' she asked.

'No, it's just me.'

'Oh, that's hard.'

There was something in her voice – was it pity? But I looked to her face and saw no judgement.

'It's hard even when you do have a partner, though,' she said and smiled. I caught a glint of something sharp hidden beneath her words.

I looked into the pram at Quinn's eyebrows which were raised comically while he slept. Would it always be like this, answering these questions? And also, what had I denied him? I would give him the world. But I hadn't given him a second parent.

At the mucky canal where the ducks drifted past with their ducklings, Chloe and I turned to go our separate ways. As I walked down the street, in my milk-stained active wear, pushing my pram, I probably looked like any other mother – one with a partner or husband or wife at home waiting.

Like so many people, my life had ended up at a different destination, at a place I'd never conceived of travelling. Despite the differences between us, I felt accepted by these women. Chloe and I were becoming friends. Even if we fell out of touch, I would be bonded to all of these women and their children for life by having met during these wild infant days.

At home, while Quinn slept in the car seat on the floor and I tried to shovel in dinner with my parents before he woke up, I took a deep breath. 'So I was thinking that Quinn and I should probably go home soon.' My parents nodded. 'Okay,' Mum said. It was resolved. I would leave in a week.

On a day of ceaseless summer rain, my dad drove Quinn and me home. 'Eternal Flame' played on the radio. Dad kept up a sweet patter with Quinn who was always on the brink of hysterics during a car ride. 'Can you see all the cars? Cars?'

Quinn made a gurgle. 'That's right, cars!' Dad said as though his grandson had cracked a quadratic equation.

When we arrived home, I found my backdoor wide open, swinging in the wind after a rainstorm. Had my subletters left it open? Quinn started grizzling. My dad was impatient to go. 'Wait,' I said. I frantically searched through the apartment, but everything was still in its place – no sign of intruders.

Quinn was screaming now. I sat down and tried to unhook my bra as a cloud of mosquitoes drifted off an indoor plant. How would I juggle unpacking the bags and the wailing baby and the mosquitoes, which needed killing? How could I do this, alone? 'Please don't go, I need your help.' I sounded desperate. I was.

Dad went out to get bug spray and, an hour later, the mosquitoes were specks on the floor and Quinn was sucking at my flesh, feeding quietly. We were alone, at last, as golden hour streaked through the windows. I could do this. I had to. I would. I must.

Double Witness

The next few months were a series of slightly blurred images – as though someone had wiped a thumb across the lens of my days.

A street corner. Outside the post office, having to breastfeed perched on a backless bench. A muslin wrap that kept falling off my shoulder to reveal my plump, naked breast. An old school friend walked past. She stopped and smiled. 'Good on you,' she said. For doing this on your own, she meant.

I nodded, trying to listen as she talked but could only feel the blister on my nipple, like a rusted nail being scraped across my skin as Quinn suckled. The breastfeeding was going well, in that he was doing it constantly and he was gaining weight. They were the markers of success. The almost mastitis, lumpy stones in my breasts that I massaged in the shower, the fact that he refused a bottle so that I could never leave him, the doctor taking a needle to scrape at the blister – which was called a milk bleb, a bubble of milk trapped under my skin – none of that mattered. The breastfeeding was going well. Mostly I enjoyed it, the rush of sleepy endorphins I got in the middle of the night, the satisfaction of his mouth sucking and sucking, like a baby vampire pulling the nutrients and goodness from my body. Like all of it, those months with my love, my darling, my boy, were streaked with pure ecstasy – like a light plane trailing a plume of smoke across the sky, beautiful one minute, spiralling to earth the next.

An ink-black night image. I was trying to change his nappy in the dark, so as not to stimulate him with the light. I heard a pop as I opened his nappy – a small, hard turd had flown across the room and hit the wall. I started to laugh, putting my hand over my mouth as I crawled around in the dark, trying to find the little shit.

Another image. Sitting on the kitchen floor, slumped against the oven, the fan drowning out his crying as I watched the timer on my phone climb to three minutes. Going into the room again and lifting the heavy cot up and down with both hands, in a rocking motion as he screamed. In and out of the room. Up and down. In and out. Up and down. In and out. Up and down. Until finally he slept. I stared at his little hands flung up by his face, his arms bent as though he was doing a gymnast's pose to show off his muscles, his fingers curled, his balding head tucked into his chin, his mouth closed in a serious line.

When I wasn't staring at my son's face, I scrolled through the WhatsApp feed from my parents' group. There were endless, inane threads about which dummies to buy, and frantic messages about sleep settling and questions about eczema, cradle cap, reflux, latching, naps, faeces, allergies, motor skills, cracked nipples, breast refusal, snot suckers, fingernails.

I realised I'd entered a secret club. It was as though a woman had appeared and pulled back a brocaded, threadbare curtain. *Come in*, she said. Behind the curtain were all the mothers. They were everywhere. The whiskered old woman at the bus stop who smiled at my baby and talked about her grown-up children. The blank-faced woman behind the checkout who transformed into sweetness when she played peekaboo with Quinn. My mother's friend who brought me bags of hand-me-down onesies and said, 'Good God, those first months are hard.' Before I had a baby, I hadn't known this club existed. Now I was part of the secret society of mothers, I saw that we were legion.

I was no different from these mothers until Valentine's Day, when a picture appeared on the thread: a crayfish and champagne brunch that a husband had laid out. The gleaming shells and talon claws served over a white tablecloth spiked a red fury in me. Then self-pity. Then self-loathing. For wanting the overstated worship that women were lavished with on certain days to make up for being taken for granted the rest of the year. Then again, was occasional worship better than none? Or was that the lie that kept women striving? Or was I merely letting my envy get the better of me when I knew nothing of this woman's husband and his daily actions?

I muted the WhatsApp thread.

Most days I got on with being a solo parent. Being a mother required continuous action, which was helpful for avoiding comparison. And while I could compare my life to others', I had no lived experience of mothering any other way. There were mutterings from the other mothers – frustration at their partner's laziness or ineptitude. That I was spared. I rarely felt despair or envy – except for that occasional jolt, the crayfish claw stabbing me in the gut.

A moving image. We were taking the bus to visit my parents. My hands gripped the pram as we hurtled down Punt Road. Quinn let out a long, constant squall. A woman sat at the front of the bus, in a short skirt over torn stockings, her lipstick in a clown smudge across her face. A sex worker. I knew this because she had yelled, 'I'm a prostitute,' as she got on the bus.

As Quinn wailed, the woman started to crackle and swear, jerking around in her seat as though she was about to pop out the window. 'How could you bring your fucking baby on the bus?' she shouted. 'You don't take a fucking baby on a bus.' That *fucking baby* she said over and over. The fucking baby kept crying. I jiggled the pram desperately, willing him to shut up, willing her to shut up, wishing I owned a car. No one moved or said anything. Another woman across the aisle smiled at me apologetically, her closed lips turned up. The baby cried and cried and cried. 'What kind of mother brings their fucking baby on the bus?' the woman declared before mercifully getting off at the next stop.

'Is he a good baby?' people wanted to know. But what was a good baby? He slept like a dream most nights, except for the weeks when he didn't. He was cheerful and beamed at passers-by, as soon as he could sit upwards in the pram. Except for when he got tired and began to wail. I'd find myself miles from home, along the beach path, the flat sea mocking my cajoling, sweating self as I half-ran home to avoid a full-scale meltdown in public. He ate well – as long as it was from my breast and not from a bottle, which meant I could only leave him for an hour or two.

Was he a good baby? He was a great baby. He was making babies great, again. Which is to say, he was a baby and he was mine and so I could see no fault in him. Because what I felt for him was operatic and vast. I loved him with a split-open tenderness. It was a Grand Canyon of love; if you got too close to its edge, you glimpsed an eddying darkness of desire-pain-terror-hope in the gulf below.

Another image; again, a view from the floor. How many days did I spend on the floor? At child height. Having a baby brought me closer to the earth, curling inwards and downwards, flattened into a lump of devotion and exhaustion. So many minutes at ground's eye view, worrying whether I was doing enough tummy time, providing enough stimulation, singing enough, talking to him enough.

I leant on the floor against a sideboard and watched as Quinn, in blue cotton overalls dotted with white flowers, lay on his stomach on the living room rug. His neck arched up like a turtle, his legs and arms kicked up and down in place. He was trying to reach for a neon green plastic truck that was just a foot beyond him. Occasionally, he turned, as if to say, *Look at me!* and gave me a gummy grin, then jerked his bobbly head. His hand trembled, reaching. I could have watched him for hours. I did.

As I watched him reach for the truck, I wondered at the other who was absent. A man I could have walked past unknowingly a hundred times in our shared city. How odd that he was not here to see this. The donor. Quinn's father. I used the word *father* only occasionally, and I never said it aloud. I didn't think of the man that way. But as much as he wasn't Quinn's father, it could also be argued that he was his father.

I wasn't ready to find out who the donor was; to face whatever unknown creature hid beneath the cot. But were there other children out there like Quinn, who shared his DNA? Who had his same wide forehead, piercing blue eyes and tufts of curls behind their ears? If I wanted, I could reach out to the IVF clinic to do what was called a 'family audit'. This would tell me how many children had been born using the same donor. It would tell me if Quinn had siblings.

A family audit. As though our children were items on a tax spreadsheet. Should I find out this information? I was curious. And more than anything, I wanted to be jolted out of the boredom of my infinite infant haze.

As Quinn's face burrowed down into the rug, I opened my laptop and clicked on my email. I typed 'Family Audit' in the subject line. It only took a few minutes to write. I hit send. I closed my laptop. I waited. I watched my son.

Quinn pushed his legs straight up on a diagonal, as though he was about to do a bunny hop. He let out an 'Ah ah!' then slid back down and inched his hand closer to the truck.

Surely, when he was born, a reverberation, like a sonar, sent out waves across the city to alert his blood kin? His possible siblings. His father.

Did this man's body know, even if his mind knew nothing of his son's existence?

How could he not? How could he not want to witness Quinn flippering his legs and arms on the bright yellow rug – swimming while staying in place? How could he not want to watch this instant of his child's life, and the next and the next? As I watched Quinn's neck strain upwards, it was unbearable. All that he was missing.

I understood when I went to an IVF clinic and bought sperm that Quinn would not have a father. *Yes, yes*, I said, signing all the legal forms. I understood that I was paying for a man's life matter separate to the man. I understood that the man would not be there to see and admire and tumble down a deep well into a never-ending, fathomless love for this baby whose dimpled hand fluttered closer to the truck. I understood that the man in question did not want to act as a father, to do as a father, to be a father.

I hadn't understood. I hadn't understood at all. I hadn't understood that on some days it would feel like indifference.

I hadn't understood that I'd have to be a double witness to my son. A mother and a father. That I'd have to store the image of my son's hand finally clasping the truck and pulling it towards himself, a grunt of glee coming from his body. 'You did it!' I said, a froth of delight bubbling up inside me, as though I'd witnessed my boy run a marathon, split an atom, cure cancer.

I hadn't understood that I would have to hold every flicker and grasp and turn of my son's life inside me twice.

Babies Bring Luck

In February 2020, at play group, our five-month-olds were lying on the floor squirming and attempting to roll. We mothers sat collapsed on blue couches under fluorescent lights surrounded by an assault of primary colours: toys and a plastic ball pit and cheerful posters: *Join the Dads' Group Sunday Fun Days!* We were trying to finish our lukewarm cups of tea: but kept being interrupted by feeding and changing and rocking.

'It's spreading across Europe,' a mother with wild, anxious eyes said as she distractedly wiped down a giraffe chew toy. 'I'm keeping my oldest son home from school for the first few weeks of term.' Chloe and I caught each other's expression and tried to mask our shared doubt. Surely the news would turn out to be a big fuss about nothing.

A few weeks later, in early March, I pumped breastmilk and put on a clean top that didn't unbutton for breastfeeding and crowbarred myself into black jeans. I was going to my first post-baby meeting about work. I was meeting a producer to discuss a TV pilot I'd written before Quinn was born. It was yet another project in my hodgepodge creative career that I'd worked on when I wasn't surviving by copywriting. My dad arrived at the back door and Quinn broke into a grin and the two of them gurgled at each other through the glass. I rushed around and listed instructions about nap times and nappies and bottles. 'Yeah, yeah,' Dad swatted me away. 'You do know I raised three children?'

In the café, the producer approached my table smiling but she was hesitant about hugging me hello. She had just arrived from being on set, filming for a TV show.

'My parents think it's a big fuss about a cold.' I shrugged.

'I don't think so. Things are getting serious overseas, they're thinking about shutting down filming so some of the actors can get back home in case they close the borders.'

I shook my head, unable to comprehend this and we turned to talk of work, of screenwriting.

I felt a dormant creature inside me wake up and stretch with the thrill of ambition, with the pleasure of making things. As I dashed out of the meeting into the rain, I was, for a glimmer, something other than just a mother.

A few weeks later, the autumn weather arrived and felt like fear on my bare legs. From the end of March, it was decreed that we were only allowed to leave our house for a few hours a day. Police patrolled the paths by the beach; yellow tape was ringed around playgrounds as though the city was dotted with crime scenes. The back fence of my building that was penning us in had turned a dirty grey that reflected the pallor of the sky.

I walked in the morning with Quinn down to the sea. A white yacht fluttered by. It was a perfect day. Joggers and cyclists and families were out as though it was any ordinary March. Quinn was tired, he had refused to nap. His small cherubic mouth was yawning. He began to let out a gradual whine and I knew I had to hurry back before the screeching wail started.

At home, he made high-pitched squalling noises of discomfort that could be teething or tiredness or being a baby. He refused to sleep and cried and cried until he'd worked himself into a ceaseless braying. I went in and out of his room a hundred times then finally breastfed him to sleep, lying on my side on the bed.

I stayed still, not wanting to move in case I woke him, and refreshed the emails on my phone. A friend in New York had sent me a photo of a bridge in Central Park that she walked to each day on her one sojourn out into the world. *This is the bridge where I pray*, she wrote. They had set up a tent hospital in Central Park and makeshift morgues around the city where I'd once lived.

We were confined to our houses and our neighbourhoods, and the shops were shuttered. While in the background, panic hovered, my days were outlined by boredom and brightness. I was still charmed by the plastic clutter of books and toys on the side of the baby bath, the proof of my son's existence; by the way he danced and kicked his legs against the highchair and smeared mush across his face during meals. As I pegged his onesies on the clothesline, I marvelled at the smallness of this person who was my person. That I'd brought him into being. I loved that his smile stopped people on the street. I loved lying on the ground, tilting his warm weight side-to-side on my chest as I sang, 'There were three in the bed and the little one said, roll over!' He giggled and giggled. He was my gladness. Every time he beamed at me, I was filled with an ecstatic life force.

In the afternoon, Chloe showed up with her pram to drop some lentil soup at my back door. She stayed outside and we told each other stories and laughed to ward off the strangeness of our new days. My parents arrived a few minutes later to take Quinn out for a walk and my dad insisted on playing us a cheesy YouTube sketch spoofing the US president. He cranked his phone to a high volume in the backyard. 'Dad,' I hissed. 'People will hear.' I was nervous I'd get in trouble for having visitors, even though they were outside.

Later that day, I got an email from the IVF clinic.

I am writing to provide you with the information you requested about other families which have been created using a clinic recruited sperm donor.

    Family 1 – Male, June 2019

    Family 2 – Male, September 2019 (This is your family)

    Family 3 – Female, December 2019

I read the email twice. There were two siblings. A boy and a girl born only a few months before and after Quinn. I felt disembodied.

Quinn, my one and only, was not a one and only. I looked at Quinn then looked away, feeling the room quiver, disoriented. He'd been diluted somehow, rendered less unique.

I remembered a movie I loved as a child starring Shirley Temple called *The Blue Bird*. The film was a strange fantasia: in one scene, a group of future children waited in a cloud-misted heaven to be born. Were there more children hovering between heaven and earth waiting to join my son's family? How many would they number? The ten-family limit now seemed huge – there could be as many as eighteen siblings if each family had two children, maybe more.

The next morning, I found an angry note taped to the front door of the building. It was handwritten and highlighted in yellow. ONE VISITOR PER PERSON OR A $1600 FINE. Suddenly every shutter and window in the building was an eye and we were being watched. At the supermarket the shelves were ransacked. I shoved a lone bag of spinach into the bottom of the pram and dialled my mum. The shock of nothing on the shelves had unseated me and I started to cry.

'What's happened? What's wrong?' I could hear the alarm in her voice.

'Quinn's fine, we're fine. It's just, what if something happens? What if you and Dad get sick? What if I get sick? What will happen to Quinn?' I was walking down the aisles now, openly sobbing.

'Oh, darling. Do you want me to come over and cook dinner?'

I snuffled out a yes.

When I got home, I ripped the note off the front door of my building and threw it in the rubbish.

Mum arrived and made a delicate chicken broth. 'Can you do this every week?' I asked. I was only half-joking. She smiled but didn't respond.

The next day and the next and the next, I circled the park with the pram, around and around and around. I counted the minutes till bedtime. I longed to be able to sit in a café and make random small talk with strangers and talk to other parents in the library and in the play centre and to hold myself together with all the incidental social threads that bound a new mother's sanity. This experience we were having of isolation was not unlike being a new mother – suddenly confined to a narrower life of domesticity. But now, that life had been whittled down even further. Behind the eyes of the masked mothers on the street with their prams, I saw a glazed darkness.

As a solo mother, I had to ask for help more often than I would have liked to, more than I was comfortable with. The asking felt like an imposition. The possibility of rejection was worse. Being refused often felt more painful than asking. I carried the legacy of family discomfort about being a burden. The belief in self-sufficiency. Now, almost weekly, I had to put my shoulder to the boulder of this discomfort and ask.

So, I asked. I practised inching the boulder aside again and again. I asked for babysitting time from my brother Tom and my parents so I could flee my apartment and bike my way along the sea and breathe the briny air. I asked Lucie to take Quinn for a walk in the pram so I could have an hour to write.

While my family and friends were generous and often helped without hesitation, that didn't make the asking or receiving simple. I felt a mix of guilty relief and queasy emptiness when Quinn wasn't there. I often imagined scenes of disaster or worried about burdening others. I could spend an entire solo jog visualising Quinn leaping from his pram into traffic or infuriating his minders by wailing for an hour.

I scrutinised the occasional glance between my parents as evidence that I was demanding too much. I imagined my friends rolling their eyes when they received a text asking if they could take Quinn for a walk. I ruminated over whether my relationship with my parents and my brother had been reduced to a transaction over my son's care.

But I asked. I had to. When the lockdown briefly ended, Chloe agreed to watch Quinn so I could take a Zoom meeting. Chloe sat on her living room floor with Quinn and her daughter Greta, while I shut myself in her study.

I was, thankfully, offered more screenwriting work on the Zoom call. The ambitious creature in me stretched further. Although, of course, I would have to find a way to fit work around mothering. I hung up and listened to Greta and Quinn babbling down the hall and wondered at this confluence of fortune and fear that had appeared six months into my child's life.

There was a saying that *babies bring luck*. It was something about the act of creating a person; that creation bloomed forth in the world and brought about other opportunities. Not only that, but the government had announced a JobKeeper payment to keep people afloat, and as I was on unpaid maternity leave, I qualified. This meant I could stretch my maternity leave further than I'd planned before I returned to my copywriting job. It was an odd silver lining that the crisis had provided the paid maternity leave that women needed.

Babies bring luck. But what was this new and dangerous world that I'd brought my son into? What fate was I tempting? My worries were interrupted by my son giggling in the next room with Greta.

Quinn spent so much time with Greta that she was almost like a sister. But she wasn't his blood kin. Did that even matter? Was blood so important? I wondered where Quinn's brother, his sister, were at this moment. Whether he would ever meet them.

I could place Quinn on the voluntary register that allowed donor siblings to connect, but there was no requirement that parents register their children. If they ever surfaced, or were forever absent from his life, what friendship and loss and hope was yet to unfold between them, my son and his siblings?

When I had told my dad about the siblings, he had said, 'Better to stay out of it.' As though there were something distasteful about finding these strangers and their donor-conceived children. But I knew that I would put Quinn on the voluntary register. I had read that it was important for a donor-conceived child's identity to connect with their siblings. Not only that. We had spent so many months drifting out to sea, separated from others, from kin and friends, from those we loved. I would try to find the rest of his family. No matter how long it took.

Sun, Milk and Moon

Sitting on the couch at night, I scrolled the newsfeed on my phone. I wandered to the fridge. Opened it. Out of milk. One lockdown had become two. Winter had unfurled into spring. Quinn's first birthday had passed by and we were still confined to our homes. Each night, whether or not the city was shuttered, I was confined by Quinn sleeping in the next room. The 7-Eleven was just down the street but I couldn't leave to buy milk, not just because my son might cry without solace. I couldn't leave, it occurred to me in a panic, because what if I stepped off the kerb and a car hit me? Then he would be left alone.

What had happened these last few months had taken a fat black pen and underlined my singleness. Each day I watched the ripples of isolation make their way across my community of solo mothers on our Facebook group. The women posted memes and messages about the loneliness of yet another lockdown. Solo mums, I'd noticed, were organised to a fault, so we commented with consoling phrases: *There's no way we could have planned for this.* We were more alone than we were before, more alone than we'd imagined was possible.

Because I was alone, I had to weigh the daily risks not just to Quinn but to myself. When I was on my own, I debated whether

I should ride my bike along the road, or drink a glass of wine that might give me cancer down the track, or run an orange light in my car? I risked all the dangers of being alive, knowing that I was the sole protector of my son.

I thought of the solo mum's Christmas picnic I had been to last year. Mara had indicated her head towards a solo mum chasing her toddler in the playground. Around the woman's head was wound a bright silk scarf. 'Terminal,' Mara said. I swallowed and looked into Mara's eyes. She shook her head imperceptibly as if to say, *I know.* The sky was blindingly blue but for a long breath, a cloud hung over us, as we contemplated the unspeakable.

I opened and shut the fridge door again to confirm that there was still no milk. From his bedroom, I heard Quinn coughing. His small lungs mucked with fluid. My radar was attuned to his cough – it felt its way along the walls of the apartment as I listened. I cocked my head to home in on his breathing. Should I check on him? No. I couldn't spend my precious free hours watching him sleep. He just had yet another winter cold.

As I made these kinds of decisions, I sometimes imagined a courtroom drama, where my child had died in hazy, tragic circumstances (it was too painful to flesh out the details). In this courtroom, a lawyer pointed at me, monologuing about my negligence to a jury.

This mother heard her son coughing YET she didn't check on him.

Or when I ran out to get bags of groceries.

This mother LEFT her child in his highchair so she could find chocolate in the boot of her car.

Or when I had a shower while Quinn was lining up his plastic trucks in the living room.

It was more important for this mother to CONDITION her HAIR, ladies and gentlemen, than to keep her child safe.

Being a mother was to live with a constant script of internal and external judgement. It was impossible to measure up. To be a good mother, I had realised, was an arbitrary standard that refused definition and was continually shifting.

In the morning, there'd be no milk for Quinn's breakfast. I weighed the options. Live in fear or live without milk? In a flash, I made a decision. The 7-Eleven was two hundred and fifty metres down the street. It was 9 pm and Quinn rarely woke up at night. I would test how far the baby monitor stretched beyond the apartment. I had bought a sound-only model because it was cheaper and I reasoned that I didn't need to watch my child at all times. Now I regretted not getting the video monitor.

Before I could second-guess myself, I threw on my coat and grabbed my keys. I gently shut my front door, clutching the monitor in my hand. Out the front door of the building with its familiar *slam*. I power walked down my driveway and onto the street towards the 7-Eleven. The monitor emitted a green glow. I listened intently to the womb sounds that whooshed through the speakers as I hurried along the footpath, past a ripped leather couch someone had thrown onto the nature strip, past the bus stop with its *Lost Cat* poster that Quinn always pointed out, past the art deco apartments that sat in hulking silence.

I thought of Mara, who had devised a system with her mother. She had explained it to me: 'So if I need nappies or milk or ice-cream – kidding,' Mara said. 'If I need nappies, and Rose is asleep, and I need to go out and get them, I text my mum that I'm going out to the shops quickly. Then if Mum doesn't hear back from me in fifteen minutes to let her know that I'm back home safe, she calls me. If there's no answer, she'll come over to my house straight away.'

Halfway down the street, the monitor at my side, a woman passed me and glanced in my direction. *She knows*, I thought. *She's seen the monitor and she knows I'm a terrible mother*. I could see the headline already: *SOLO MOTHER ARRESTED FOR CHILD NEGLIGENCE*. The monitor cut out. I could see the 7-Eleven, its bright lights were a beacon glowing less than fifty metres from where I was standing. I would be in and out. But I couldn't do it, my anxiety was like a helicopter propellor, my head was about to lift off.

I turned around and half-ran back to my apartment – my bra-less breasts thudded under my jumper. The sound of the monitor hissed back to life.

As solo mothers, we were the sun and the moon and the milk for our children. My worry for Quinn was only eclipsed by my worry about what would happen to him if I was gone. I scurried back down the driveway and slammed the front door shut.

Inside, I opened Quinn's bedroom door in slow motion so I didn't wake him. He snuffled loudly, breathing through his mouth. How was it that I was solely responsible for this child? It was terrifying.

As I stood in his doorway, I had to fight the instinct to turn and look for someone behind me. To find the person who would steady my fall, to locate the adult in the room, as reassuring as dusk and daybreak. But there was no one else here. I was the adult now. I was the mother. Each second, each minute, each hour, I was his only parent.

I watched as Quinn threw his fist in the air and curled and uncurled his fingers in sleep, scratching at an invisible tiger. Then my body returned to itself and the terror was gone.

How Do You Do It?

'So I asked Simon to take the washing out of the machine. And he does. But he just dumps the wet clothes on the couch,' said Chloe, as she forked noodles into her mouth like they might be taken away from her. Everyone at the table groaned in recognition.

Our children were now eighteen months old, and my parents' group was having a rare dinner out at a Malaysian restaurant without said children. The table was piled with noodles and glasses of red wine and we had reached shrieking pitch to hear ourselves over the one toddler present who was fussing in her mother's lap at the end of the table. 'I had to bring her because my husband still can't manage bedtime,' the woman said with a sigh. Another woman picked up the empty wine bottle and held it aloft trying to catch the waiter's attention.

'Simon doesn't do bedtime either … and never gets up in the night when Greta wakes up,' Chloe said. The wine-bottle holder, who hadn't had a full night's sleep for almost ten years between her two children, deadpanned, 'I've got three children: my son, my daughter and my husband.' The waiter arrived and she handed him the empty bottle. 'Another one, please.' So polite, the way we women were.

In cis-hetero couples, it wasn't news that women still did more household work, even when both parents worked full-time. This was worse during the lockdowns. In May 2021, the stats showed that women were almost twice as likely as men to have spent twenty or more hours a week on unpaid caring and supervision of children.

The table of mothers was electric with frustration. I pressed the button on my phone to see if my brother Tom, who was thankfully doing his share of unpaid babysitting, had texted to say that Quinn was awake. No messages. I exhaled and tuned back into Chloe speaking.

'I'm basically doing it on my own too.' Chloe looked at me. 'In every way, except for bedtime.' I smiled and didn't point out that her husband was earning an income, that she could split all her bills with another person, get family discounts, afford to buy a house.

I had returned to work when Quinn was a little over one year old. I had found a new copywriting job with a female manager who was warm and empathic and understood what motherhood entailed.

I had weathered the anguish of those early months – the screaming, clinging day care drop-off and the hurry to the office and then, at day's end, back again to pick him up. I had also started writing this book part-time and after hours. There were days when I felt like my selfhood had been ground down to a paste but I reasoned that many mothers felt the same way, single or otherwise. There were always other parents – those with children who were sick or who had special needs – who could put my complaints to shame.

And I didn't mind Chloe's words that she was doing it alone because, at that moment, I felt relieved: I had no partner to help me at home but also no one to resent.

The next morning, Quinn and I were in the foyer of our building. I was trying to stop him from yanking the leaves off the wilting succulents in pots under the stairs and get him into the pram. 'I don't know how you do it,' my Chilean neighbour said as she came down the stairs, balancing her ten-month-old on her hips. Her child stared at us with his solemn eyes. 'Seriously, how do you do it?' My neighbour shook her head. I smiled and shrugged.

A few days later, Mara and I were eating a late dinner of cold burgers with red wine on a weekend away down the coast. We'd lugged travel cots and strollers and all the incidental baby items that made a trip away with children more work than holiday. Mara's face was pale; she had spent almost two hours lying next to her toddler waiting for her to drop off to sleep. 'People always say it to me too. "How do you do it?" And it's like, do you really want to know how I do it? Now I just say, "It's hard." Because it is.' Mara sipped her wine.

'Why is it that "I don't know how you do it" never feels like a compliment?' I asked myself as much as Mara.

'It's like they want you to reassure them, to make them feel better,' she said.

'Or they're warding off the possibility of disaster that they could end up living our lives,' I said.

We smiled. Gallows humour.

Of course, there was enormous physical labour in parenting alone but the irony of parenting solo was that I couldn't do it alone. American author Mikki Morrissette had coined the term 'Choice Moms' in 2005 in the US to describe solo mothers. She wrote, 'The goal of a single parent is not to raise our children alone. The goal is to consciously create the village in which we and our children will thrive.'

My family, who had their trepidations about me choosing solo motherhood had surprised me with their generosity, their presence, their time. My dad had retired a few months after Quinn was born and he split his time between helping raise Quinn, playing golf and boring his friends with photos of his first grandchild.

Once a week, when I was at work, my dad picked Quinn up from day care. 'How's my boy?' Dad grinned as Quinn disentangled himself from the sandpit and trucks and ran towards him. He hoisted him up in his arms, kissed him on the cheek and took him to my parents' home – feeding him gingerbread cookies on the way. There, my mum played with Quinn, voicing the wooden figures of his train set in a high, funny voice that he adored.

My parents knew the push and pull and lift and cajole. Weathered the whine. Kissed sticky cheeks. Listened to *more more more*. They wiped away dirt and blood and snot and shit and dribble from soft cheeks, hands, bottom. They fed and bathed and threaded his legs and arms into onesies so that when I arrived from work, he was cotton soft, clean and fed, hair brushed and ready to be taken home to bed.

On Saturday nights, once he was old enough, Quinn often stayed at my parents' house overnight so that I could go out.

'Gwampa! Gwampa!' Quinn yelled when he stood up in his cot in the morning. It was Grandpa who made him Weet-Bix and changed his nappies and took him on scooter rides to the park. My dad was the ballast to my son's life.

My mum was the medical professional who was always on call. On days we didn't see my parents, I FaceTimed her to consult on bruises and fevers and rashes. 'Hmm.' Mum squinted into the phone at Quinn's chest which was covered in pimpled dots. 'Looks like a viral rash. Nothing to worry about. It'll clear up.' My mother's calm when it came to medical issues and her knowledge of the International Classification of Diseases were what every new parent should be gifted with when they left the hospital with a baby.

The staff at day care also knew my brother Tom. He arrived every week, an anomalous twenty-something in a long black coat, with a shock of bleached-blond hair, lankily striding in like a delinquent Brit punk absconding with a small, delighted boy. When I arrived home, my apartment was a mess of dishes and Duplo. My son was raised mid-air as Tom pretended to be a crane, trumpeting a loud mechanical sound from his mouth. Quinn giggled hysterically and yelled, ''Gain! 'Gain!'

Babysitters and friends and neighbours gave me bric-a-brac-ed hours that let me work and kept me tethered to the adult world.

Of course, some days, I still hoped for a partner to step in. But there was a radical secret that no one told you as a girl, when you were taught to dream of marriage: having a partner didn't necessarily make your life better. But we were supposed to find wholeness in a pair. As though we were dolls that magically flickered alive when another person took us in their arms.

꩜

I arrived home after day care pick-up, hauling four large bags and a cumbersome plastic toy bus as I herded the zigzagging figure of my toddler inside. We opened the back door, to let the autumn breeze air out the place. Quinn hurtled between the small yard, where he pushed an old heavy metal trike around, and then abandoned it to run back into the living room, beetling his Matchbox cars along the windowsill.

I fried meatballs and listened to the Beach Boys, as the afternoon sun reflected off the orange brick apartments across the street. *Bluey* played on TV ('Mum! Dad!' shouted the opening song cheerfully) as my son half-watched, running in and out, dragging his *storm* (stool) to the bench and shovelling meatballs in his mouth. 'More, more, more,' he yelled and I squirted tomato sauce onto his plate. He climbed down and did some happy jump twirls just for the hell of it, just because he was alive.

I kissed the top of his head, sticky curls askew, as I moved between the stove and the bench – and then to the bathroom where I ran the bath while Quinn played in the living room. My heart lurched whenever I heard an unseen thud. In the bathroom, we chanted through the ritual of undress: 'Arms up! Pants off! Top off!' He obediently lifted his arms up and I pulled his singlet off to reveal his small rotund belly, the miniature butterfly wings of his shoulder blades.

I sat by the bath as he squirted water out of a blue plastic crab onto the tiles. We played a game which involved cupping my hand into a tunnel perched on the bath's edge, which he whizzed the cars through. When the water was stone cold, I cajoled him into extracting the plug, and lifted his soapy body out of the bath.

'Wanna be cosy!' he demanded as I wrapped the towel around him and rubbed dry the creases of his knees and neck and face. Curled up in a towel, he put his arms around me and we stood for a long moment in a hug, as I swayed my body a little from side to side, feeling his small chest (thin blue veins from ribs to belly) breathing against mine. Then he broke away, flinging off his towel and I chased his naked body around the apartment and wrestled his flippering body into a nappy, singlet and onesie.

I read and re-read *Hairy Maclary* (''Gain! 'Gain! 'Gain') and *We're Going on a Bear Hunt*. When it got to *Thomas the Tank Engine*, I made up the story to avoid the boredom of treacly morality and pages of dense type ('And then the Fat Controller and all his cronies decided they weren't employing enough women, so they hired a female CEO!'). Quinn sat curled in my lap, head bent over the book, his mouth shut in a serious line of concentration.

On the way to the bedroom, I fielded a tantrum about wanting a cracker with Vegemite and a demand to turn on the 'Tee Bee'. I prodded a toothbrush into his mouth, which he ejected, and it smacked against the wall. I picked him up and he wriggled in protest as I carried him to the cot. 'Wock like a baby! Wock like a baby!' he yelled. And so I rocked him in my arms and sang 'Rock-a-bye Baby'. I incorporated a comedic lunge, pretending to drop him when the cradle fell. It always got a laugh.

In his cot, he rolled over and curled onto his stomach. 'Stawy! Stawy,' he said. So I told him a well-worn story about a little boy and a whale whooshing him to see his uncle Nick in Sydney, where they ate ice-cream (this had to be repeated a minimum of three times). On a good night, when I was lucky, I patted him on the back, said, 'I love you, time for sleepy byes,' and closed the door on the thudding white noise.

That was how I did it.

But that was not the answer you were looking for, was it? The answer was not a productivity spreadsheet or 'How to do less while doing more' or 'Here are the top five ways to multitask like a mom-boss!' You wanted to know how I lived through the tireless banality of parenting, how could a person be, what was her very essence, her core, when she was almost always with her child?

One answer was that I often found myself staring at my boy – his startlingly blue eyes, the baby fat curve of his cheeks, his cupid's bow mouth always open, a long line of drool hanging from his chin, his curls that corkscrewed behind his ears then fluffed out from the top and sides of his head like young Einstein. I could stare at him all day. His beauty. His constant movement. His adult body in miniature.

When he laughed it was as though the sound was gurgling up from a happy well. When he travelled, he ran, arms held out, barrelling towards everything that life had to give him. The pleasure I got from observing him, from being with him, from his seriousness and his coyness and his hammy-ness, his him-ness, was ecstatic and unending.

The other answer was that parallel to this pleasure, there were minutes and hours and days that were like being stretched out on a rack – as time elongated me so that my body was a taut wire of anxiety and exhaustion. When the motherness of me felt unceasing and suffocating – that my sole self without an echo, an other, a reprieve, surely couldn't sustain us both until bedtime.

But who ever said anything about parenting being pure bliss? I had read that parents were less happy but they felt like their lives had more meaning. It was an answer that could bring comfort to us all – those with children and those who were childfree.

Like all parents, I told myself that having my child felt like destiny, a miracle that I would recount to him one day: *You were made in this year in history, on that summer day, when this sperm had the good fortune to hit that egg.* This destined person, for whom I bent my being to keep alive, gave me purpose. A purpose both sacred, and shit smeared, all at once.

Cargo

A few months after our mothers' group dinner, I stood in the playground, clasping and unclasping my hands to warm them against the cold tongue of wind from Antarctica. I was staring at a dad in a pair of cargo pants adorned with numerous baggy pockets. He was pushing his daughter on a swing that let out a grating metal squeal each time she arced into the air. I counted the pockets on his pants. Could I love that man? The pants were bad, but I could look past it. I looked at his daughter on the swing, snot streaming from her nostril to lip. Could I love her as my own?

I was slightly tipsy on cold margaritas that Chloe had made. Now that the lockdowns had stretched into another year, another winter, it was our weekly tradition to have late afternoon Monday cocktails on our day off from our paid jobs. Chloe had spared nothing – bringing salt and lemon to top our travel cup margaritas. I watched her pour the premixed drink from a thermos into the cups with elegant precision.

'You used to work in a bar, didn't you?'

She laughed. 'Is it that obvious? I was a very good bartender.'

'Of course you were.'

We drank from our cups as the wind whipped away our fragments of conversations and we ran in opposite directions to collect our toddlers. Our children were always centimetres away from tipping off the edge of some stairs or running smack into a metal pole.

'Simon moved out a few months ago,' Chloe told me, darting her eyes away from mine.

Chloe was guarded, she had kept this to herself.

'Oh no, I'm sorry,' I yelled as I ran towards a slide that Quinn stood atop in his puffer jacket, a cracker in one hand, about to fall down face first. He saw me, and decided to leap towards my arms instead. I caught his padded body and it almost slammed me to the ground, then he quickly shimmied off me and ran back to climb the steps.

Chloe's daughter, Greta, was dragging her to the slide, holding firm to her hand.

'It's okay, it's been coming for a long time. We've been in counselling for almost a year and nothing's changed,' Chloe called back to me.

Chloe's eyes were wide, dark ringed.

'A friend of mine saw him on Tinder. I know we're not technically together anymore, but it was a knife through the heart.' She laughed. I sipped on my drink and shook my head.

Our masks were hanging from our ears now, our hands frozen from holding our drinks. Both of us were slightly unhinged from lockdown: greedy for conversation, talking too fast, feeling mad from being stuck inside with our children for another winter.

'What's going to happen with Greta?' I looked at Chloe's pale, solemn daughter who was sitting at the top of the slide, unsure about the descent.

'We're still trying to figure it out ... I tried to talk about custody. I basically have her one hundred per cent of the time but Simon said to me that that would be a matter for the family court.'

The wind knifed through me at the mention of family court. I looked down at Greta, her dark eyes were fathomless. I had known her since she was a tiny baby.

'My counsellor told me to have a bag packed, in case,' Chloe said.

'In case?' I was trying to thread this together. Chloe's handsome husband who had been so polite and engaging when I met him.

I turned to find Quinn had disappeared with Greta – we heard the sound of their muffled giggling and spotted the tops of their heads weaving through some scraggly bushes behind the play equipment. Laughing, we retrieved their wriggling bodies and lifted them protesting into their prams.

'I often think about you, on your own,' Chloe said as we wheeled through the park. 'What you're doing is easier.'

This wasn't the first time I'd heard this statement from women in relationships. I was never sure what I felt or how to respond. Should I refute the idea? Should I accept it as a compliment? Should I feel smug and vindicated?

Only that morning, in the hallway of my building, the sensor light had snapped off. Quinn was running up and down as I tried to put his bike helmet on when we were suddenly plunged into the grey dark of morning. For him, it was a hilarious game. He ran to my bike and yanked the wheel, and I watched as the heavy bike tipped towards him in slow motion. I lunged and caught it just in time. Even though he was safe, I still saw the reel of disaster play out: the fall and crush of his small body.

Being a solo parent was crazy, I thought, as I knelt on the floor in the hallway of the building, trying to force the helmet onto his head. Quinn yanked his head away, wailing and crouching against our front door. Immediately guilty, I tried to rewind the thought – as though it would whisk my son away. The collision of intense love and chaos was not something I wanted to will away. But these toddler mornings often called for two sets of hands.

Talking to Chloe, who was staring at my life wistfully, I'd changed my mind about the madness of solo parenting. We said goodbye and forked off on our separate paths home. As I pushed the pram underneath the bare elms, I thought about Chloe and her husband. Good looking, smart and successful; owners of a house in one of Melbourne's blue-chip suburbs. All I could see was their skeleton outlines; their beloved baby caught between them.

There had been other women I knew, single, separated mothers who dropped their voices and slid their eyes away as they catalogued all the varieties of violence they'd felt, physical and otherwise. I tried not to think about the statistics on domestic abuse and male-perpetrated violence.

As I walked home, the spindly trees glowed in the winter dusk and the cocktail dulled the edge of everything to make it magic. I was *that* mother, the one who was tipsy in the early evening, but it had made me slow and contemplative. I suddenly had all the patience in the world for Quinn, who was yelling, 'MUM-MUM-MUM-MUM-MUM,' at top volume, just to hear his own voice. I pulled his jacket hood over his fluffy curls and he broke into shrieks of annoyance.

We passed by a couple with a pram with a new baby sleeping inside, bundled under layers of blankets. I noticed they were both holding cups too, no doubt filled with wine or stiff liquids as all of Melbourne was doing. The couple were staring ahead stony faced, as they silently wheeled under the darkening sky to wherever they were going.

Full credit to the couples – the ones who had children and still managed to be kind and loving and present for one another. Perhaps I didn't have the graciousness and good humour to raise a baby with someone else: the drudgery, the boredom, the silences, the domestic chores, the long nights and the in-betweens. To live with the itching of resentment that eventually built to breaking point. All of that holding onto togetherness once the grenade of a baby had been thrown into a couple's midst took a quarry's worth of grit. Maybe the couples were the real heroes in all this.

So many of them hadn't made it through those first few years of parenting to reach the other side. A study in the UK found that one-fifth of couples broke up in the year after they had a baby.

Chloe had embarked on a destination, a partnership with a man that led to a baby. She had found herself in a dark wood, the road lost to her. What comfort could I give her? I was supposed to tell her she'd find someone else. But I didn't know if I believed it.

I embarked upon what I hoped would be Chloe's destination – making a family with a partner – but had been rerouted to a family of my own making. It was a choice borne of circumstance but also to guard against unhappiness.

I was relieved I didn't have to contend with the pain of separation. At the end of each day, for better or worse, I only had myself to blame. At the end of the day, I had no bitter ex to negotiate with, no one to take my son from me. He was mine alone.

I thought of all the men in cargo pants. Not yet, not today. Today it felt safer just the two of us, making our way home at sunset; the clouds inked purple, while the couple walking in the other direction became a blur, indistinguishable from the night.

Song of a Single Girl

'What do you think happened to Dave?' Lucie asked me as we took our second lockdown walk for the week around the park. The leaves mulched into yellow mud under our shoes and Quinn sang an off-key song to himself. Lucie wasn't the first to ask. For some reason I found the question irritating; as if my life still needed to be measured in relationship to my ex, to a man.

'Have you ever thought about getting in touch with him?'

'No, not really.' I avoided Lucie's eyes.

I had thought about contacting him. I had no wish to rekindle a spark or a friendship, but occasionally, I remembered our intimacy. How strange it was that we could go from sharing the very oxygen someone breathed each night, just millimetres away from us in bed, to never speaking or touching again.

A few times Dave's ghost had appeared on someone else's social media feed. I saw his rapturous smile in a church pew at a friend's wedding in New York or a blur of half his face and elbow raised on a dance floor. These photos sometimes lured me down into the treacherous tunnels of the internet. There I found a Christmas photo, his family sitting on some steps outside in woollen sweaters, posed together and grinning. A woman I'd never seen before sat behind Dave on a step. She was a ruddy-faced redhead who looked like she enjoyed hikes and crocheting and making pea and ham soup. She had her hand on his shoulder but it was balled into a fist. I thought I could see a glint of something on her left ring finger. The air was knocked out of my body for a second and I quickly pressed the phone screen to black.

As my heartbeat slowed to normal, and the hours passed, I started to feel oddly affectionate towards this woman and all the things she hoped for her life. I hoped they would come true. Not because I was a good person. But because she was my avatar going forward into a future with Dave.

⚘

In the evenings, when Quinn slept, while all the windows of the restaurants and bars were still dark, still closed, I mindlessly scrolled through Facebook. I stumbled on a post from a woman in a single mothers' group I belonged to in the US. It went something like this:

Today, I am finally leaving this group. All our dreams have come true. I'm getting married to a wonderful man. God knew what my baby girl and I needed and now we've found him.

The comments poured in.

Congratulations! I want that for myself one day too.
How wonderful! I hope I meet someone.
Amazing, go get it!

I muted the group for thirty days. I didn't begrudge this woman her happiness but what annoyed me was the subtext that she'd been emancipated. That she'd been freed from her terrible predicament as a single parent – because she'd arrived, she'd been chosen by a man who could rescue her from all this.

I felt conflicted. On the one hand, there were days – and long nights – when I wanted saving. When I could use another pair of hands to parent. I pendulumed back and forth, unable to decide if coupledom was what I wanted or needed.

The myth of being saved was bred in me. My formidable mum still believed in the myth of male knighthood. 'There goes your knight in shining armour,' I'd tease Mum after Dad had aggrieved her by committing one of the many sins of marriage, like leaving a room mid-argument or buying the wrong-sized grocery bags. I was, childishly, trying to score a point for the a-romantics, for the single mothers.

The single mother on Facebook who was getting married had chosen to go at motherhood alone – some would call it a confident and brave choice. Sure, her life was filled with a complexity that I could never guess at, and her arrival at marriage may have felt heaven-sent – especially in the US which didn't have the same social security for single mothers. But I sensed that she believed that ours was a compromised route, one that we ultimately needed saving from. That we were the outcasts. The ones who had been picked over and chosen last for the basketball team. Love's failures.

Heterosexual women who chose marriage – and children – were exulted and sanctified. Single, childless women were not. So many of the rituals of life were around babies and weddings: the showers and hens' nights and ceremonies and parties.

Don't get me wrong, I didn't eschew love. But why was romantic love given such weight over every other kind of love? As Esther Perel said, historically, when our worlds were smaller, we used to look to the village of people to give us all the different shades of love we needed in our lives. But modern love placed the emphasis and end point for love onto our romantic partner, which was, she argued, an impossible burden for relationships to live up to.

⚭

There was a song that had been an earworm in my head for over two decades. I first sang it when I was fourteen, standing on the proscenium arch stage in the dusty school hall, wearing a classic '90s brown corduroy waistcoat and blue shirt over my baggy jeans.

The piano dutifully played in a steady, laborious beat, counting me in. In a pure, strained soprano, I sang into a handheld microphone:

> *This is the song of a single girl*
> *Nobody's sweetheart*
> *And alone in the world*
> *Waiting for someone*
> *Honest and true*
> *Waiting for someone*
> *Who … will whisper I love you*

On either side of me, in a straight line, stood a chorus of girls in unflattering calf-length skirts, blue shirts and dicky bow ties and, inexplicably, a girl in a head-to-toe dalmatian outfit. The girls were doing limp choreography in sync, hula-ing their bodies as though they were Hawaiian dancers. At one point, they waggled their fingers in accusation at me for being 'single and alone'.

Then, out of nowhere, the chorus of girls burst to life, singing in an off-key, high pitch, schooling me in the realities of married life: the unhappiness, the endless washing of nappies, the unceasing domestic work, morning and night.

I heard the audience of parents laughing in recognition as I acted out these scenes of domestic misery. Then I rejoindered with my finale verse. A revelation. No longer a 'hopeless cause', or just an unloved 'wallflower', I'd woken up to 'this masculine world'. The song ended with me vowing to remain single.

Now, over two decades later, when I watched the blurry camcorder footage of this performance, I felt fond of this girl singing – some version of me a million shed cells ago in her pubescent body. And I felt a flush of embarrassment. Not for her strained voice or stiff acting but because it had revealed a truth to myself.

Perhaps the song, which I still hummed in the shower, had shaped my life, setting me on a course to forever 'stay a single girl'. Had my teenage feminist outrage at the inequities that women face calcified over time into an unconscious decision? Did I believe it was better to be single?

Maybe I'd actually chosen this path all along.

American writer Kate Bolick wrote about the 'spinster wish' she felt throughout adulthood, even as she found herself in and out of relationships. While the word spinster, she explained, had become a slur, it didn't used to be – it was merely a description of a financially independent gal in good old fifteenth-century Europe who spun thread. Bolick's spinster wish was to be alone and unfettered. Even though, she stated, heterosexual women were duty-bound to organise their life around the fact of who and when they would marry. Women who must live, she wrote, in a constant, tiring state of anticipation that love would appear out of nowhere.

By the time I arrived at solo motherhood, I was tired of this state of anticipation. Of dressing for love's arrival. (*Don't wear those saggy-arsed tracksuit pants to the supermarket!* an inner voice reprimanded. *You might meet the love of your life by the bananas.*)

In all the pre-baby years of dating, each time a possibility appeared, I'd found myself entering that state of early romantic madness. I became distracted and agitated. I second-guessed every word the other said, while feigning casualness and sitting elegantly with my head tilted just so, to catch the light at a flattering angle. I stared anxiously at the ellipses of messages being written; I gave my loyalties over to people I barely knew.

Anticipating and embarking on love was a constant state of unease that was supposedly balanced by the sweetness of romance's rewards. But to let love go? To defect from the quest? Surely, that was spinsterish. That would admit some kind of brittle defeat.

And what was a life without romantic love, without risk? Was stepping aside from love a way of standing on the sidelines of life? Didn't I want a soaring, heart-stopping, operatic kind of love? If it existed.

At dinner one night, a married friend lowered her voice and turned to Lucie and me. 'So tell me, are you dating anyone?' she asked.

'Lucie, are you dating anyone?' I volleyed the question to Lucie, trying to keep my face straight. She shot me a loaded look. The friends around us went quiet, their eager faces leaning across the table.

Coupled people meant well. I knew they did. Or they wanted to live vicariously through my dating life. They hoped against hope for my happiness. But underneath it all was the feeling that I must fall into line – to march in step in my designated pair. That the world was flooding with shit. And we needed to hop aboard the boat, two by two.

Why did I need to be dating someone? Why was love, a relationship, such an emblem of success? How was it that we so easily skipped past the domestic and emotional load that women carried in straight relationships and instead deemed that the partnered women were love's winners? What if I embraced the radical idea that being single was not just something that must be borne but was often far better than exhausting myself taking care of a man?

At my parents' house, as we lazed in front of the TV one night, I said to my mum, 'What are men really good for, anyway?'

I was being flippant, incendiary.

'Sex,' she immediately said.

She had a point. I didn't want to live a life devoid of touch. But now that I was on the other side of the quest to find the father of my future children, what I felt was relief. I felt spared of the endless dramas of a burgeoning relationship.

Perhaps this was something that I'd known all along – perhaps I'd chosen this solo life because of the freedom it brought.

This is the part where I am supposed to tell you to take your life by the ovaries, choose a family of your own making, run with the wolves, smear your face with the contents of your moon cup and dance around the firepit dressed like Stevie Nicks on the cover of *Rumours*.

It's where I am supposed to say that I've crossed over the threshold and that I've shed the feeling that I should meet someone. That I don't wish for another body to stand between myself and the onslaught of the world's opinion. But I still live in the world.

'But are you lonely?' asked journalist Jacinta Tynan when she was interviewing me for a story on single mothers. 'All the single mothers I spoke to said they were lonely with and without their children, it was a common thread.'

The question gave me pause.

'I'm less lonely than I was before I became a mother,' I answered. 'When I was looking for someone to have a family with.'

I was lonely sometimes, usually on Sunday mornings when the fathers gathered at the playground while the mothers were sleeping in and I fell into the trap of compare and despair.

But mostly, when I was with my son, I felt like my heart was firmly rooted in my body, flushed through with life. Was I lonely? To some, I might be incomplete as a single person. I could only conclude that I was both whole and in pieces. I was not chosen, nor had I chosen another. I was wholly fine with that.

As Lucie and I circled the park again, we wound past the flowerless stems of the rose garden where couples got married each spring. 'Have you ever thought about getting in touch with him?' Lucie had asked. She was still looking at me, waiting for my answer.

What would I hope to get from communicating with Dave, my last true love? What good would it do to open that door?

I'd composed sentences in my mind: *Hope you're well … I have a son now … He's donor conceived because, well, you know how men won't commit to baby making.* Maybe I'd add some laugh-crying emojis.

I tried to imagine his reply but it was a blank. I didn't want to know if he was engaged or married or had children of his own. Perhaps because those things still had the power to wound me. Mostly because it didn't matter. It didn't matter what he was doing or who he loved or whether he was a father. I wished him happiness, but his life no longer touched mine.

As I picked up Quinn's woollen beanie that he had piffed onto the ground and tried, and failed, to put it back on his head, I said to Lucie, 'I know the world is weird right now but I'm so much happier since I've had Quinn.'

It felt almost taboo to say it, in a world that places a premium on coupledom, but I was happy. Where did one put this happiness in a society that thought a single woman was a dangling thread? I was free and unbound, which others saw as both dangerous and titillating.

Lucie nodded. 'I know. People keep asking me, "How is she?"' She mimicked their hushed tone, their curiosity and concern. 'And I tell them that I've known you for twenty years and you're the happiest and most grounded I've ever seen you.'

Daddy

When I walked into the pub, the light was golden and the air crackled with end-of-lockdown release. I was at a Christmas dinner with old friends. I caught sight of a guy I used to know across the table. He was tall and stooped, with a cheeky grin. *Hi*, I mouthed. He smiled back. We hadn't seen each other in a few years. He was in my extended circle; a guy I'd gone on a few dates with years ago that never went anywhere. Just another blip in those pre-child years of turbo dating to find a baby daddy.

Halfway through dinner, I turned to find him sitting next to me. He had deliberately moved to make his way to my side.

I turned to him. 'Are you having a post-lockdown existential crisis like everyone else I've spoken to tonight?'

'I'm always having an existential crisis.' The guy laughed.

We talked and laughed, and laughed and talked. I remembered how funny he was and how much of a man-child too, unable to cook or drive or go to therapy even though he admitted he needed it. As he took a hit of his vape and complained about his ex-girlfriend, I realised I was doing something I hadn't done for a long time. Flirting.

It seemed impossible that I was still desirable. First there had been the transformation of matrescence, my body softening and loosening and being split apart. Then after birth, I had become a thing, milk bloated and weighed down, no longer an object of desire. This was followed by two years of isolation which had put the world of human contact behind glass. Romance was a fiction that I consumed on a screen or a page. It was no longer something that happened to people in real life. I couldn't feel the edges of myself anymore, I was separate to my body.

Nine months earlier, when Quinn was eighteen months old, I'd risen to the surface of a dream. A dream where I was constantly swaddling and being suckled at, more animal than woman. As a mother, my identity had been obliterated and reconstituted a million times in the last few years. But waking up from that dream, I found that my creative ambitions and desires crackled and flamed back to life.

So, I'd got back online and resumed swiping. I'd felt a familiar frustration as I scrolled through blurry profile pics and muscle shots of naked torsos and selfies shot at murderously unflattering angles. *No single mums*, a few men wrote in their profiles. *No, no, no, no*, I swiped. I went on a few dates that didn't lead anywhere but felt like good practice, a way to shed my mother self and play at sitting opposite a man with a drink in hand.

Later that night, the guy and I were playing pool. We were having a good time when he ruined it.

'I'm scared of kids,' he admitted as he potted a shot effortlessly. 'I'm fine when I've got a book or something to read them. When the material's already prepared.'

I laughed but something inside me crumbled.

I hadn't realised it until he said those words that, despite being happily single, I'd been carrying a wish. Sure, it'd be nice to meet someone who was romantically interested in me. But more than that, I wanted to meet someone who would love my son. I could picture it all; as saccharine as a Sorbent commercial: flashes of someone tossing my son into the air as he giggled, someone holding my son's hand as he jumped over the waves, someone wiping the grime off his upturned face.

I had been hoping that before my son was more than a baby and less than a boy-child, a magical father would arrive. Don't misunderstand me, I wasn't avoiding telling Quinn about his origins. He was familiar with the literature that *Love Makes a Family*, and that families come in all shapes and sizes. Even though our family didn't have a daddy, I fortified him against this fact by listing and lining up all the people around us like soldiers (grandparents, uncles, an aunty, cousins and friends).

I had also read, more than once, a study that soothed me. It found that the 'presence of two parents – or of a male parent – is not essential for children to flourish' and that, rather than family structure influencing a child's happiness, the real factor was the quality of family relationships.

I followed VARTA's recommendations that you should tell your donor-conceived child from an early age about their origins, in language that they could understand. Each night, before bed, when Quinn rolled over onto his stomach and I pulled up his blue woollen blanket and patted the small of his back, I told him a story about a woman who wanted a baby so much that she went to the doctor and got a seed from a nice man. The doctor put the seed in the woman's tummy and then a baby grew and grew. One day the baby was so big that it had to come out. He was born and she named him Quinn, I declared (a revelation that always made his eyes open wide). And the baby made the mummy so happy.

At the library, I skimmed through children's books to veto those with only heterosexual families and father protagonists. Sometimes I changed *Daddy* to *Mummy* as I read aloud – ruining the satisfying rhyme in certain stories. I strived to find a delicate balance, not erasing fathers from stories so that I didn't present parenting as an endeavour of mothers only.

At day care pick-up, I stood with Quinn as two big-eyed toddlers lingered by us, waiting for a crumb of my attention.

'My daddy is coming,' a blond boy told me solemnly.

'*My* daddy is coming,' echoed a boy with perfect lashes.

I watched Quinn's face for any reaction.

I realised I couldn't guard him against this. I hadn't anticipated the talk of *daddies* that were part of the shriek and cacophony of each day with other children.

There was the other side of it too. In my orbit there were both coupled and solo dads who fielded questions and assumptions about the presence of a 'mummy'.

I felt relief when I found other parents who didn't fit the paradigm. Despite what you saw on TV, we were legion. The 2021 Australian census still asked for the 'mother' and 'father' of a child to be listed. Despite its blind spots, the census did show that more than one million families were helmed by a single parent.

'Where's his daddy?' a young girl side-eyed Quinn and me at the playground as she used her leg to spin the merry-go-round at a dangerous clip. Despite confidently stating that my son was donor conceived to adults who asked, she had caught me off balance. As I watched her spin faster and faster, I sifted through possible answers. Instead of an absence (*Quinn doesn't have a daddy*), I wanted to affirm what we did have (*In our family, we have a mummy and uncles etc.*). But that answer made me sound like those parents who wrung teachability from every moment, giving sing-songy speeches from the lectern of adulthood.

It also avoided the question and, by doing so, outlined a father-shaped hole. If I didn't state the obvious – *there is no daddy* – was my avoidance casting a shadow of shame behind the true answer? The word donor required explanation, especially to a child.

We were still remaking the terms for how these unseen men fitted within our families. And until the binary of male and female parents wasn't assumed to be present in every family picture, single mothers and fathers and queer couples would always be answering some variant of, *Where's Daddy/Mummy?*

Where was his daddy? What parts of him were mine and what parts belonged to someone else? So often, strangers and friends and family told me that Quinn looked like me. When I looked at his face, sometimes I felt like I was staring at an echo, a memory of myself. Each time someone pointed out the resemblance, I felt satisfaction but also relief. Lucie had once asked where Quinn got his dexterousness from. I shrugged and said it must be the donor. 'Ahh, it's from his daddy,' she looked at my son lovingly. The word 'daddy' grated but I didn't correct her.

There were nights when I stared at Quinn sleeping in bed and didn't recognise his slack-jawed face. Was it the donor I was seeing in his expression? When he pushed his favourite yellow digger around, I wondered whether he would be left- or right-handed, and which one of us, or his ancestors, he would take after.

Where's his daddy? The answer was in his face, his movements, a map to which I didn't have all the keys.

The girl on the merry-go-round was still looking at me, waiting for an answer. Her whirling was making me dizzy.

'He doesn't have a daddy,' I said in a flash. Quinn didn't blink.

In the pub, the windows were now turning dark and the room was reaching a drunken pitch. My friends were starting to slur so I waved goodbye to everyone. I was driving, smugly looking forward to tomorrow's lack of hangover while parenting.

At the bar, I saw the guy I used to know, waiting to order another round. I said goodbye, hugging him.

'By the way, Ally.' He put his hand on my arm. 'You look really great.'

A white-hot flush ran through me. I started to walk to the door. 'And Ally,' he called out.

I turned around to catch what he was yelling across the room.

'It'd be really great to see you again.'

Now that I had a child, if I chose love, I wanted to be with someone who was an adult. Someone who could meet me where I was at, who was firmly rooted in their life – their solid branches reaching towards me. I wanted a person who could cook me dinner, who could be a co-parent and partner amid the chaos of my days. The bar for what I wanted in a partner had risen as the stakes of what I was responsible for had too: the love and steady happiness of my son.

As I watched the guy's hopeful face across the pub, I was tempted but I could see that what he was holding out to me was a life I had left behind. He belonged in the past where I could have risked being caught up by a capricious and unknowable heart. Where I was willing to nudge and cajole and lug a man's needs along. Now, it wouldn't be enough. I waved and walked out the door into the uncomplicated summer evening.

Don't Stop

A few weeks later, on Christmas Eve, Quinn and I were down the coast with my family. I hung my wet bathers up on the line and puttered into the open-plan kitchen. It was cocktail hour and a lazy glisten coated the house. I could see Mum on the couch playing Words With Friends on her phone, drinking a G and T. I veered around Dad emptying the dishwasher in the kitchen to get to the wine glasses. My brother Tom was on his laptop at the dining table.

Outside, Quinn was trampling the grass on a stars and stripes patterned trike he liked to circle in and out of the house. On the bench, I scrolled through my phone until I found Fleetwood Mac's 'Don't Stop' and pressed play. Those piano chords and the ramping drumbeat started up. I turned it up and I shook my way into the living room. 'Come on!' I yelled to my family. Mum looked surprised but she was, as always, the first to join in. She stood up from the couch and did a wobbly shimmy, arms held straight out like she was balancing dinner plates. She pulled a fish-face in a half-sexy, half-silly send-up of herself.

Dad kept emptying dishes but managed a little shoulder shake and a head bop. Tom raised his arms in the air in a punching motion but kept his eyes on the screen until I hopped over to him and dragged him out of the chair. Then he danced like a DJ scratching two mini turntables, hands close to his body. Quinn clattered inside on his trike and took us all in. When he saw me, he put out his hand like a police officer stopping traffic and yelled, 'MUMMY, DON'T DANCE! DON'T DANCE.'

He ran over to me, but I grabbed both his hands and dipped him up and down. He giggled and fell onto the carpet and wriggled around on his back like a turtle trying to right itself. Then I took Mum's hands and we danced together, because as Fleetwood Mac sang, yesterday was gone, and whatever had passed between us, for now, was forgotten. We twisted our arms in and out. I caught her silly expression, her eyes aglimmer and I started to laugh.

My family, the ones who had been there for me all along. Steady and maddening and funny and loyal and weird and true.

Later, lying on the couch, I turned to Mum and asked her a question, as lightly as possible. 'So how do you feel about my choice now to have a kid on my own?'

Mum furrowed her brow, thinking. 'What you were doing … I was deadset against it. Deadset against it,' she repeated. 'But Quinn has brought us inordinate, inordinate, inordinate amounts of joy.'

As she said the words, a golden light poured into me. A circular light that ran through me to Quinn and back to his grandmother. The blessing of a mother loving the child of her child.

'And it's been such a gift to me that you're a wonderful mother … We're glad you did it. He's the best thing we've ever seen.'

I had spent my entire life collecting my achievements – like a child at the beach with a handful of gleaming shells, holding them up for my parents' approval. Now here was my greatest achievement, my son. He was more than a shining prize, though. In the presence of my son, my mum and I were suspended above our relationship to each other. He had given us that.

Quinn's babbling voice interrupted us as he came down the stairs, in his pyjamas, curls wet from his bath, holding Dad's hand.

'One at a time, Gwampa, one at a time,' he was saying.

'That's right, one at a time,' said Dad.

And now Quinn was running towards me, face lit up. 'Mummmmyyyyyy.'

Acknowledgements

I'm grateful to Writers Victoria for my studio at the creative hub of Glenfern. The loss of Glenfern is a huge blow for the Australian literary community – so many more books were yet to be written there.

My huge thanks to my publishing team at Hachette and beyond: Fiona Hazard for being the mother of this book; Jacquie Brown for her rigour and for always including me every step of the way; and to Alexa Roberts, Bethany Nevile, Alissa Dinallo and everyone else behind the scenes. Thank you to my wonderful agent, Sharne McGee. Some parts of this book originally appeared in the *Good Weekend* – thank you to Katrina Strickland for commissioning and believing in that story.

Many thanks to so many friends who listened to me *kvetch* and cheered me on and played a part in a million and one ways: Claire Murray, Peachie Pantelis, Marnie McDonald, Issy Raphael, Libby Butler, Sara Farrington, Mia Rovegno, Janice Maffei, Rachel Chiodo, Shelley Krape, Lindsay Ratowsky, Kris Smith, Suzy Tuxen, Georgia Benjamin and Claire Thomas.

To my generous first readers and friends for their life-changing insight and advice: Georgia Clark, Regina Lane and Declan Fay, and to editor Rose Skelton.

To all the solo mothers who gamely told me everything, some of whom didn't make it into these pages but their lives and friendships underpin this book: Sarah McBride, Maree Fewster, Laura Kenny, Jessica Little, Leanne Haynes, Michele Galea, Deepa Mylangam, Miranda Archer, Kate Windon and Clare Kelaher. Thank you to all the women who I met through the VARTA solo mums' support group and to the supportive, badass community of the Australia Solo Mum by Choice Facebook group.

To Samara Hodgson for shining a light ahead of me and being a stellar example of a friend and a mother, and to the whole Hodgson family, including Artur Brisita.

Thank you to legal guru Fiona Kelly for generously fact checking and providing insight. And to Felicity Marlowe for telling me about the history of LGBTQI+ activism – all solo mothers in Victoria are indebted to you for the work you did and the dedication of Love Makes a Family.

Thank you to John McBain, Kate Stern and Marita Voller at Melbourne IVF for being part of this book in so many ways.

Thanks to my doula, Gabrielle Nancarrow, to my midwife, Rachael Bond, and to Jenny Bell for taking care of both Quinn and me.

To my research assistant, Anthea Yang. To my Brooklyn TV writers' group for letting me take a sabbatical and for believing in me and this book – you are a constant source of support. To Cathy Grant and all at GDJ for creating a mother-friendly workspace.

Thank you to my fellow community of lovely writers at Glenfern, in particular Isabel Robinson and Stephen Sholl for the babysitting and encouragement.

Thank you to my family members, named and unnamed, for generously agreeing to be placed in these pages. To my brother Tom Collier and my parents for babysitting so I could write. To Nick Collier and Ellen Simpson for their support. In particular, thank you to my mum and dad, Robin and Neil Collier, for making me into a writer (even though they may regret it at times). And to Quinn, my one and only and everything.

This book was written on the unceded lands of the Boon Wurrung/Bunurong people of the Eastern Kulin Nation, and I offer my respect to the original storytellers and traditional owners of this land, past and present.

Resources

This is not an exhaustive list of resources, but these are some of the places and words I found along the way as I considered solo motherhood.

Online

Australia Solo Mothers by Choice Facebook Group
facebook.com/AustraliaSoloMothersbyChoice/

Donor Children Australia Facebook Group
A group created to provide support for parents of donor-conceived children. facebook.com/groups/Donorchildrenaustralia/

Victorian Assisted Reproductive Treatment Authority (VARTA)
varta.org.au

Solo Mums by Choice Australia
smcaustralia.org.au

Single Mothers by Choice USA
singlemothersbychoice.org

International Principles for Donor Conception and Surrogacy
A vital set of proposed principles about donor-conceived people's rights – which have been drafted to be in accordance with the United Nations Convention on the Rights of the Child (UNCRC). I hope all potential parents, ART clinics and lawmakers will take these to heart. donorconceivedaustralia.org.au/geneva-principles

Not by Accident, podcast, 2017–2018, Sophie Harper. podcasts.apple. com/au/podcast/not-by-accident/id1095859621

Books

Kate Bolick, *Spinster: Making a Life of One's Own*, Crown Publishing, New York, 2016.

Emma Brockes, *An Excellent Choice: Panic and Joy on My Solo Path to Motherhood*, Penguin, New York, 2018.

Nell Frizzell, *The Panic Years: Dates, Doubts and the Mother of All Decisions*, Flatiron Books, New York, 2021.

Sheila Heti, *Motherhood*, Henry Holt and Company, New York, 2018.

Ariel Levy, *The Rules Do Not Apply*, Random House, New York, 2017.

Glynnis MacNicol, *No One Tells You This*, Simon & Schuster, New York, 2018.

Gina Rushton, *The Most Important Job in the World*, Macmillan Australia, Sydney, 2022.

Donna Ward, *She I Dare Not Name: A Spinster's Meditations on Life*, Allen & Unwin, Sydney, 2020.

Sources

Act I

Next
J Updike, *Bech is Back*, André Deutsch Limited, London, 1983, p 124.

Baby Want
A Rotkirch, '"All that she wants is a (nother) baby"? Longing for children as a fertility incentive of growing importance', *Journal of Evolutionary Psychology*, 5(1–4):1789–2082, March 2007, p 89–104. researchgate.net/publication/228628496_All_that_she_wants_is_a_nother_baby'_Longing_for_children_as_a_fertility_incentive_of_growing_importance

Act II

Wrong
New York Magazine, 'Falling in love with your anonymous sperm donor', New York Sex Lives Podcast, 19 May, 2016. archive.org/details/podcast_new-york-magazines-sex-lives_falling-love-with-your-anon_1000368980304

Medical History
D Dempsey, 'Lesbians' right to choose, children's right to know', *Sperm Wars,* ABC Books, Sydney, 2001, p 186.

AAP, 'Solo Victorian women get IVF rights', *Financial Review*, 29 July 2000. afr.com/politics/making-the-news-20000729-k9j75

S Hunter, 'Urgent changes needed to halt new "stolen generation"', *The Age*, 5 December 2022. theage.com.au/national/victoria/urgent-changes-needed-to-halt-new-stolen-generation-20221204-p5c3hj.html

AAP, 'Children happier with a mother and father: PM', *The Age,* 19 April 2002. theage.com.au/national/children-happier-with-a-mother-and-father-pm-20020419-gdu51x.html

Act III

Liberation

G Callaghan, '"What makes a father?": the sperm donor who asked the courts to answer this question tells his story', *Good Weekend, Sydney Morning Herald*, 28 July, 2019. theage.com.au/national/what-makes-a-father-the-sperm-donor-who-asked-the-courts-to-answer-this-question-tells-his-story-20190722-p529js.html

Donor

Australia Backpackers Seeking Sperm Donation, About Section. facebook.com/groups/176366092996255/

Act IV

The Lonely Woman

JE Newman, RC Paul, GM Chambers, 'Assisted reproductive technology in Australia and New Zealand 2020', Australia and New Zealand Assisted Reproduction Database, UNSW Sydney, October 2022, p vii. npesu.unsw.edu.au/sites/default/files/npesu/data_collection/Assisted%20Reproductive%20Technology%20in%20Australia%20and%20New%20Zealand%202020.pdf

VARTA, Annual Report 2021/2022, p 33. varta.org.au/resources/annual-reports

Cryos International, 'Single mother by choice using a sperm donor', cryosinternational.com/en-gb/dk-shop/private/about-sperm/why-use-a-sperm-donor/single-mother-by-choice/

Act V

How Do You Do It

Australian Bureau of Statistics, 'Household Impacts of COVID-19 Survey: Insights into the prevalence and nature of impacts from COVID-19 on households in Australia', May/June 2021. abs.gov.au/statistics/people/people-and-communities/household-impacts-covid-19-survey/jun-2021

M Morrissette, choicemoms.org

M O'Gieblyn, 'Are there hidden advantages to pain and suffering?', *The New Yorker*, 15 November, 2021. newyorker.com/magazine/2021/11/15/are-there-hidden-advantages-to-pain-and-suffering-hurts-so-good-leigh-cowart-the-sweet-spot-paul-bloom

Cargo

SWNS Digital, 'These are the most common reasons new parents break-up', October 2019. swnsdigital.com/uk/2019/10/these-are-the-most-common-reasons-new-parents-break-up/

E Perel, *The State of Affairs*, HarperCollins, New York, 2017, p 44.

K Bolick, *Spinster: Making a Life of One's Own*, Crown Publishing Group, New York, 2016.

Australian Bureau of Statistics, 'Household and families: Census, 2021'. abs.gov.au/statistics/people/people-and-communities/household-and-families-census/latest-release

Daddy

S Golombok, S Zadeh, T Freeman, J Lysons, S Foley, 'Single mothers by choice: parenting and child adjustment in middle childhood', *Journal of Family Psychology*, 17 September, 2020. ncbi.nlm.nih.gov/pmc/articles/PMC8054653/

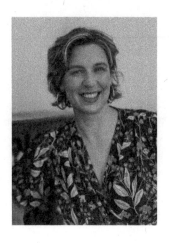

Alexandra Collier has written for theatre, screen and print. Her writing has appeared in *The Age*, the *Sydney Morning Herald* and *The Guardian*. She spent a decade in New York where her plays were produced Off Broadway, including *Triplight*, a musical written with ARIA award-winning composer Greta Gertler-Gold. She now lives by the bay in Melbourne/Naarm with her son. This is her first book.

hachette
AUSTRALIA

If you would like to find out more about
Hachette Australia, our authors, upcoming events
and new releases, you can visit our website or our
social media channels:

hachette.com.au

f HachetteAustralia

🐦 📷 HachetteAus